DATE DUE

Demco, Inc. 38-293

Hands Off
My Belly!

Shawn A. Tassone, MD
Kathryn M. Landherr, MD

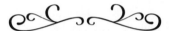

Hands Off My Belly!

The Pregnant Woman's
Survival Guide to Myths,
Mothers, and Moods

Prometheus Books

59 John Glenn Drive
Amherst, New York 14228-2119

Published 2009 by Prometheus Books

Inquiries should be addressed to
Prometheus Books
59 John Glenn Drive
Amherst, New York 14228–2119
VOICE: 716–691–0133, ext. 210
FAX: 716–691–0137
WWW.PROMETHEUSBOOKS.COM

13 12 11 10 09   5 4 3 2 1

Library of Congress Cataloging-in-Publication Data

Landherr, Kathryn M., 1966–
    Hands off my belly! The pregnant woman's guide to surviving myths, mothers, and moods / by Kathryn M. Landherr and Shawn A. Tassone.
        p. cm.
    Includes index.
    ISBN 978–1–59102–753–9 (pbk. : alk. paper)
    1. Pregnancy—Popular works. 2. Medical misconceptions. I. Tassone, Shawn A., 1967–

RG551 .L36 2009
618.2—dc22

2009019081

Printed in the United States of America on acid-free paper

To Our Mothers

Carol Ann Wetzell Landherr
1938–1999

and

Karen Lynn Bechard (Tassone)
1945–2001

Too young to leave us.

Contents

Section Three. Early Pregnancy and Mood Myths

Section Four. Second and Third Trimester Myths

Section Five. The Mythical Grab Bag—
　　Placentas, Twins, and Culture

Section Six. The Seven Habits to a
　　Highly Enjoyable Pregnancy

Acknowledgments

Nothing of this magnitude could be accomplished without the help of many people. We wish to express a great deal of gratitude toward Kathy Schlotec, NP, who held the office together during the months we were writing. Lynn Wiese-Snyed helped us start this process over a cup of coffee. A respected writer in her own right, Lynn is forever supportive, persistent, and ultimately, forgiving. We want to thank our agent, Katharine Sands, with the Sarah Jane Freymann Literary Agency; she believed in this process and found the perfect publishing house for this work. Steven L. Mitchell, editor in chief at Prometheus Books, is a true professional, and his expertise is one of the reasons Prometheus Books is a leader in health-care nonfiction.

We also would like to thank the team at Prometheus Books that made this book come to life. Christine Kramer, our production manager, has been a wonderful asset and coach in helping us give birth to this book. We want to thank Julia DeGraf for bearing with us as we learned the art of editing, and for making this a beautiful work.

C. Scott Naylor, MD, has been a friend and colleague since medical school at Creighton University. It seems like a lifetime ago, but I am so glad to have his support with this project.

Lynn Wiese-Snyed and Gretchen Kelly have added imagination, editorial prowess, and creative writing to this project for which we are eternally grateful. Both of them helped us understand the true meaning of a deadline.

Our patients are the reason this book was possible. Their questions and their pushing us for answers—often found off the beaten path—helped bring flesh to this book. We are grateful and honored that they chose us to partner with them in the birth of their babies.

Finally, we would like to acknowledge our children, Hannah, Hunter, Angelo, and Anthony. We hope this book shows them that anything is possible if you dedicate yourself to an idea and surround yourself with excellent people.

Foreword

After years of practicing as a perinatologist, there is almost nothing I haven't seen or heard when it comes to the wonderful world of pregnancy. From the country plains of Nebraska to the rowdy streets of Compton, I have been blessed with the opportunity to practice obstetrics in some of the most fascinating places in our country. Along the way, I've amassed a multitude of stories, some heartwarming, some shocking, some outlandish, and some just downright hysterical. Laughter is indeed one of the joys of life, and few things make me smile more than hearing about the various tales—and old wives' tales—related to pregnancy.

Over the past nineteen years of practice, I've heard a myriad of myths and misunderstandings about pregnancy: sexual positions during conception, the validity of Chinese calendars, round tummies, protruding tummies, carrying high, carrying low, craving sweets, having heartburn—the list goes on and on.

One of the joys of my day is showing a patient her baby for the first time on ultrasound. At their initial visit, parents anxiously await hearing their baby's heartbeat for the very first time. And often, once they hear it, the couple will proceed to break into a debate about their baby's gender based on their baby's heart rate. Fast...it's a boy? Or was it slow...it's a girl? If only Mother Nature was that easy to understand. A baby's heart-beat is, in fact, a miracle, but as miraculous as it may be, its speed has no relation to the baby's gender. I just have to chuckle because while everyone in the room is staring intently at the heart in the center of the baby's chest, one need only look a bit more southward between the legs for a much more accurate and definitive determination. If the apple has a stem, it's a boy. And if there's no stem, it's a girl.

Heart rate myths abound, but what about those related to heartburn? What on earth could acid indigestion possibly have to say about the growing baby? Well, there are a lot of people out there who swear that a mother suffering from heartburn is a sign of the baby having a solid head of hair. While I can't draw any solid conclusions on this matter, I do know that my wife had a nasty case of heartburn for the duration of her first pregnancy. At the end of nine months, much to the surprise of those in the "heartburn = lots of hair" camp, our little daughter was born as bald as a cute little bowling ball.

Yet of all the myths, misunderstandings, and surprise endings of pregnancy, my personal favorite is from a couple who didn't want to know the gender of their unborn baby. "There are very few surprises in life," said the dad, "and we want to embrace the anticipation." For the whole nine months, this couple had enjoyed not knowing. Would it be pink for a girl or blue for a boy? As the mom-to-be entered labor, the excitement grew. Dad was pacing around the hospital room waiting for the big moment when he happened to look over at the nursing paperwork scattered on a side table. His eyes locked on the fourth line from the top and read, "Gender: male." The dad was devastated. After all these long months, he had been waiting for the surprise of the big moment, and now it was ruined. But what happened next was an even bigger surprise. What the dad didn't realize was that often when nurses don't know the gender of the baby beforehand, they will write "___male" on the birth record papers but leave enough room in case the baby is a girl, in which case the nurse can simply write "fe" in front of the "___male" and easily turn the word into "female." Well, long story short, after several hard hours of labor, the baby finally made its entrance. As the dad looked on, out came the head, out came the arms, out came the legs, out came everything except the wee-wee. The dad's shock was instantaneous. "My boy has no penis!" he exclaimed. "I saw the gender written on the nurses' paperwork, and it said 'male.' What's happening?" The nurses had to contain themselves from laughing hysterically and managed to reassure the dad, "Oh, not to worry, we always write 'male' in the gender column. That way, if it's a boy we don't have to change it, and if it's a girl, we just have to add the 'fe.'" This story just goes to show us that while knowledge is important, sometimes too much knowledge—or not enough of the right knowledge—can often get in the way of a truly special and magical occasion.

Pregnancy, from start to end, is, indeed, a wild and wacky ride. When a woman embarks on the nine-month journey, she will usually come to the quick realization that everyone has an opinion to share, a story to tell, and advice to give. In fact, at no other time in her life will a woman be approached daily by complete strangers who not only want to touch her tummy but will also feel compelled to share their pearls of wisdom. Sometimes the information is sound medical advice and is worthy of taking, but most of the time, their "pearls" of wisdom are no more than grainy pebbles that are constantly shifting position in the sand.

In *Hands Off My Belly*, Drs. Tassone and Landherr have identified many of the popular myths, tales, and misunderstandings that continuously shower pregnant women. Using thorough research, personal experience, and sound medical reasoning, this book gives comfort to soon-to-be parents of what's true and what's not. But in the end, only the baby knows the real truth. And perhaps, after birth, that's why they scream so darn loud at us. Maybe, just maybe, they're trying to tell us to relax more, enjoy the process, laugh a little, and definitely don't believe everything you hear. Pregnancy is a joyous time. It's a time to learn about your body and the growing baby inside—it's not a time to let unfounded tales and advice from well-wishers sidetrack the soon-to-be parents from the real joy at hand, the surprise and wonder of their newborn baby.

C. Scott Naylor, MD
Director, Pacific Perinatal Center
Torrance, California

Introduction

As we go from room to room in our clinic, we are asked hundreds of questions every day. Many of these questions come from our pregnant patients and their spouses regarding their pregnancy. One thing we have noticed in our conversations with thousands of patients is that many of these questions have to do with myths or superstitions pertaining to pregnancy and even myths surrounding conception itself. Myths and superstitions can be very powerful, particularly for a pregnant woman, and it matters not if she is Caucasian, Hispanic, African American, or Asian. All cultures have myths and superstitions regarding the pregnant woman and her health that have been passed down from generation to generation.

It is natural for men and women to rely on myth, and this has been true for thousands of years, but what exactly is a myth? Myths are projections of our imaginations that help us make an irrational world rational. Pregnancy is a time in a woman's life that is both magical and confusing. It is no surprise that women have relied on myths to help understand and deal with pregnancy, as it is the backbone of creation, both miraculous and mystical, to say the least. Some types of mythical thinking are thought to be ridiculous and even crazy, but many of the stories surrounding pregnancy have been passed down through the ages and are taken as "the word," yet no one can explain exactly why they are true or where they even came from.

Take, for instance, the story of one of the first pregnancies we cared for when we moved to Tucson, Arizona. We will delve deeper into this tale in a later chapter, but let's use it to highlight a prime example of a pregnancy myth.

Julie is a seventeen-year-old Hispanic female and finds herself pregnant in a family with a wonderful sense of respect and support. Throughout her pregnancy, Julie is being cared for by me in the office and by her grandmother at home. During one of her office visits, as we exposed her belly to listen to the fetal heart tones, I noticed that she had made a small apron of paper clips that she had adorned over the front of her abdomen. I thought it a bit odd, but I figured maybe I was not up on the current fashions.

As we sat down to talk, I asked her if she had any questions. She looked around the room in a nervous fashion and asked me what I knew about the eclipse of the sun. We were supposed to have a partial eclipse of the sun that day, so I explained to her what I knew about its occurrence. She stopped me and said, "No, tell me what it can do to my baby and how best to stop it." Now I was really lost, so I asked her to explain exactly what her fear was. She told me that early that morning her nana had told her that there was to be a solar eclipse today and that if she did not wear metal over the baby, the baby would be born with a cleft lip. I spent the next ten minutes trying to explain to her how I was fairly certain that this would not be the case, but she seemed uninterested in my answer, and I had learned long ago not to try to out-explain a grandmother. I went to my medical assistant, a very intelligent Hispanic girl who happened to be pregnant herself, and asked her what the concept was behind the solar eclipse and the cleft lip. She laughed at the notion and told me that her mother had recently told her the same thing. I asked her if she knew where the story had originated, but she just remembered hearing it as a little girl. I asked her if she was wearing her paper clip belt. She started laughing, gently lifted the bottom of her shirt, and stuck through the belt of her scrubs was a solitary paper clip.

"Do you think one will be enough?" she laughed.

This story is just one example of the many myths and traditions we have encountered in our practice. We wanted to write this book to give back to our patients some of what they have given us. We will present the myths and superstitions related to preconception, pregnancy, and delivery that our patients have shared with us and help explain and understand their derivation from a medical standpoint.

Each chapter will include a real-life patient encounter to help illustrate a particular myth. The first chapter will provide a short discussion on myths and superstitions in order to gain a basic understanding of where they come from and how they help us organize our societies, as well as our lives. In some cases they help to formulate our belief system, and thereby are obviously important and can even be crucial to a particular patient. The goal of this book is to give the medical and factual information surrounding the myth and, in some cases, describe the derivations of these myths and discuss why they have such impact. Our goals are not to counter anyone's belief system or oppose the understandings of generations of women. We merely want to present the material in a way that will help our patients, and hopefully others, to understand the interesting and sometimes amusing myths that surround the pregnant female and serve to make the pregnancy a more rich and full experience.

Throughout the book there will be footnotes to guide those who desire further reading regarding certain topics. We believe there is nothing more wonderful than an informed patient and an open-minded physician.

Kathryn M. Landherr, MD
Shawn A. Tassone, MD
Tucson, Arizona, April 2009

Section One
Superstition and Myth

Chapter One
Superstition and Myth

Myth: a popular belief or tradition that has grown up around something or someone; *especially*: one embodying the ideals and institutions of a society or segment of society.

Superstition: a belief or practice resulting from ignorance, fear of the unknown, trust in magic or chance, or a false conception of causation. An irrational, abject attitude of mind toward the supernatural, nature, or God resulting from superstition.

It is natural for a book related to the different myths and superstitions of pregnancy to discuss what makes a myth and why societies have developed them; what makes a superstition and why we practice them.

Humans have been involved with myth since before there was organized language. Creating myths has always been a way for people to cope with and make sense of their surroundings. Even in the twenty-first century, when we no longer need to hunt or gather, we still need to understand life. We continue to rely on myths in this day and age not so much to survive physically but to survive spiritually. Mythology is based in rituals. Rituals keep us on a certain path by pure repetition and familiarity. When a woman becomes pregnant for the first time, she is entering a new chapter of her life, an unfamiliar one. This new chapter can be overwhelming and can cause feelings of inadequacy, as well as fear and excitement.

Myths are usually drawn from a life or death experience, and pregnancy is certainly considered a life experience. Occasionally we field questions from a patient that may seem somewhat strange, like "Will I deliver my baby this weekend because it is a full moon?" However, many of these questions are more than likely the remnant of some mythical story from many centuries past that at one time was more detailed and complex. A myth is not a story told for its own sake; it shows us how to understand our world and how to behave in it.[1]

When we look at pregnancy, we see that modern medicine has removed many of the rituals and replaced them with the more up-to-date office setting and delivery room. Today we have a much better medical understanding of the birth and death process and thus we no longer have as much need to create myths to understand these concepts. We do, however, live in a society that places increasing demands on our time and makes us ever involved, or uninvolved, in the life experience. We really do not have the time anymore to just sit and feel the baby move or wonder about the mystical process of being pregnant. I think it is a fundamental human thought to wonder where we came from, and even when the answer may be literally sitting under our noses, we are simply too busy to understand it. Our ancestors, however, were very concerned with the process of pregnancy and created mythical stories to help them cope with their experiences. For instance, in medieval times a pregnant woman who had a stillbirth was thought to have conceived the child out of wedlock and was therefore being punished. People in those days lacked the medical knowledge to realize that the infant actually had a fatal birth defect and it was not the mother's fault at all.

In this book, and in our society, we use the word *myth* to define something that is most likely false but helps us look at something in a certain way. We speak of a myth as something that has been confabulated. We have to understand that myths in the truest sense are not based on fact. In the example above, the explanation of a stillbirth was not thought of as a myth but rather as a universal truth. Reason and knowledge enter the human psyche and it becomes clear that the myth is not plausible, but we can still wonder "what if" and thereby create a superstition.

A myth is true because it is effective, not because it gives us factual information. If, however, it does not give us new insight into the deeper meaning of life, it has failed.[2] In the example above, the myth involved placing an ethical standard on sexual relationships of the time. If people thought they would be punished for having sex out of wedlock, then perhaps they would be less likely to do so. In this example, the myth works as a way for that society to establish boundaries in its world and possibly bring order to a chaotic situation.

In our current day, and in our modern clinics, we have come to realize that trying to grapple with myth and superstition is not easy and at times is better left alone. Science and medicine will replace myths in the Western world, in some ways, unless we all continue to perpetuate them. Life would be much less interesting without our myths, for they are the stories we heard as children; the fables our grandmothers told us as we lay in bed in twilight sleep.

The Salem Witch Trials are an example of an apocalyptic time in human history when myths were challenged by scientific fact. Many of the myths surrounding women and the devil resurfaced, and individuals involved thought they had the science available to prove whether these fears were true. Our goal here is not to try to convince the patient that the questions she asks have a right or wrong answer, for they are what they are. We want to delve deeper into the origin of the question and figure out what each patient fears in order to understand the patient better and hopefully help her more. For example, why is she afraid that reaching over her head will wrap the umbilical cord around the baby's neck? We also feel it is our duty to provide patients with the most accurate information and let them come to their own conclusions. We jokingly stated earlier that we had learned not to argue with grandmothers, but this is no joke. Many families are structured in a matriarchal pattern, and we have no desire to convince a patient that the beliefs of her familial leader are false, for this could undermine her feelings of family as well as the good that the myth was trying to achieve.

Superstitions are those practices that we avoid in order to avert some sort of bad luck or ill will. Sayings such as "step on a crack, break your mother's back" seem meaningful when you are a child, but once you test this superstition and it does not hold up, it no longer has you in its grasp. Superstitions have even entered the labor and delivery unit at our hospital. We currently have twenty labor and delivery rooms, but the last room is numbered "21," not "20." This is because there is no room number 13. Haven't you noticed that many high-rise buildings do not have a thirteenth floor? Many mothers would be reluctant to have their baby in room 13 of a labor and delivery unit. Do any of us even remember why the number 13 is considered unlucky? More than likely we do not, but the fear is strong enough that a hospital would not number a room 13. Interestingly enough, the reason for unlucky 13 originates in the history of the menstrual cycle. One of the early calendars was the lunar calendar that had thirteen 28-day months. These 28-day lunar cycles were consistent with the normal menstrual cycle. The 28-day calendars were used by peasants, while the Church was utilizing a different solar calendar that had only 12 months. In general, the matriarchy was associated with the number 13 and the night, while the patriarchy was represented by the number 12 and the day. As our societies changed from a goddess structure to the Christ model, the number 13 was demonized. Fear of the number 13 grew to such heights that people were afraid to even speak the number out loud. As a result, we see such terms as "a baker's dozen."

As you can see, superstitions are associated with a behavior, or an aversion to a behavior, in response to a certain myth. They are rampant today and at times are just as powerful as they were hundreds of years ago. There are also many superstitions that have survived even though the meaning behind them has all but disappeared.

Notes

1. Karen Armstrong, *A Short History of Myth* (New York: Canongate, 2005), p. 4.

2. Ibid., p. 10.

Section Two

Infertility and Conception Myths

Chapter Two

Infertility Myths
Planting a Seed

Y ou've been trying to get pregnant, but month after month you seem to be coming up empty. Well-meaning friends and family have started offering advice. Stand on your head after having sex, suggests your cousin. Chill out and relax, says your best friend. Adopt a baby and you'll get pregnant, advises a coworker. So, what are you to do? Infertility affects 15 to 20 percent of couples. Are you and your partner one of those couples? Most infertility issues can be successfully resolved with help from reproductive endocrinologists, but there are couples who, despite trying every advanced technology for infertility (and perhaps, out of desperation, every myth and superstition out there), just cannot have children. Luckily, this percentage is small. In this chapter, we'll sort through the myths, superstitions, and science associated with infertility.

1. If we can't get pregnant, it's my fault.

Before either partner takes the blame, you should know that 40 percent of infertility is attributable to the woman and 40 percent is attributable to the man. The remaining 20 percent probably relates to a problem that involves both of you and therefore is harder to pinpoint. It's easy to play the blame game when it comes to infertility, but we recommend avoiding it because it only adds to the stress already present. It seems like simple advice, but we'll give it anyway. Instead, support each other as you attempt to resolve any problems.

The main causes for female infertility include the following conditions:

- Endometriosis

    Over five million women in North America have endometriosis. It occurs when endometrial tissue—the tissue that lines the uterus—becomes implanted in portions of the pelvis where it doesn't belong. It can implant anywhere, but the ovaries, fallopian tubes, uterus, and colon are among the most common sites. The symptoms are as varied as the patients who have the disease. Many women experience no symptoms other than infertility, while others may have diffuse pelvic pain, pain with intercourse, and painful periods. The degree of pain is not related to the amount of endometriosis present in the patient. Studies indicate that about 20 percent of women diagnosed with endometriosis cannot conceive without medical intervention.

    If you have endometriosis and are having difficulty becoming pregnant, it could be that your fallopian tubes are partially or completely blocked. Your physician may recommend a surgical procedure to open the tubes. If your tubes are open but aren't effectively transporting the egg, then you might consider an assisted reproductive technique (ART) such as intrauterine insemination (IUI) or in vitro fertilization (IVF). The IUI technique involves using medication to stimulate the development of multiple eggs and timing ovulation. Your partner's semen is then implanted during ovulation into your uterine cavity through a hollow tube the diameter of a coffee straw. In IVF, your egg and your partner's sperm are fertilized in a lab and then transferred to your uterus. Usually through one of these methods, endometriosis-related infertility can be overcome.
- Ovulation Problems

    During ovulation your ovaries are stimulated by a certain hormonal milieu to release an egg. It occurs midcycle and is the first step in conception. Ovulation is essential in the regulation of menstrual periods as well as conception. Hormonal imbalances can result in certain conditions characterized by extremely irregular ovulation or lack of ovulation. A woman with polycystic ovarian syndrome (PCOS), for instance, will have difficulty conceiving due to irregular ovulation and irregular periods. Other common symptoms include excessive hair growth, acne, and weight gain.

Another hormonal issue is the overproduction of the hormone prolactin, made by the pituitary gland. Prolactin naturally increases during breastfeeding and plays a role in preventing pregnancy in women who breastfeed their babies during the first six postpartum months. If this hormone is elevated, it can cause irregular or absent ovulation.

Ovulation can also be affected if thyroid hormone levels are too high or too low.

Generally speaking, issues involving anovulation (no egg production) can be corrected. In the cases of polycystic ovarian syndrome, women can be placed on Metformin, a drug used to treat diabetes. It helps regulate ovulation by helping regulate insulin levels. These women also may take the drug Clomid, which can help stimulate ovarian follicles to release an egg. If you are diagnosed with either increased prolactin production or thyroid irregularities, consult an endocrine specialist, who can recommend an appropriate treatment. Once these issues are corrected, ovulation and menstrual flow will become normal.

- Blocked Fallopian Tubes

   Multiple treatments are available to correct tubal factor infertility, which can result from endometriosis, pelvic inflammatory disease, scarring from previous surgery, or, in rare instances, congenital factors. Tubal factor infertility is usually diagnosed by an outpatient radiology technique called hysterosalpingogram (HSG).* Dye is injected into the uterus and tracked with an x-ray as it flows into the fallopian tubes. The dye will accumulate in one spot if there is a

---

*An HSG is a radiological test performed either at a hospital or a radiology center. Radiopaque dye is pushed into the uterus through the cervix. This dye then fills the uterine cavity and eventually pushes out into the fallopian tubes. With normal open fallopian tubes the radiologist will see the dye spill into the pelvic cavity. This is a common test for infertility, and while you may experience mild to moderate cramping, the test is of short duration.

blockage in the tube. Treatment for this type of infertility can involve surgery to remove the block or an assisted reproductive technique such as intrauterine insemination or in vitro fertilization, as described above.

• Cervical Factor Infertility

Here, the infertility problem most likely involves a problem with the mucus in your cervix. The mucus could contain anti-sperm antibodies that destroy your partner's sperm once they enter your cervix. This situation can be diagnosed by performing a postcoital test* at your doctor's office within two to four hours of having sex with your partner. There, a cervical mucus specimen will be obtained and the mucus will be evaluated under a microscope for the presence of viable sperm.

If all of the sperm in the specimen are dead, further testing may be required to determine why this has occurred. A sperm penetration test, for example, checks to see if sperm can move through cervical mucus; an anti-sperm antibody test will check for antibodies that destroy sperm once they enter the cervix. If there is a problem with cervical factor infertility, it usually can be resolved by intrauterine insemination as described above.

2. We've been trying for over a year and my partner says it's not his fault.

As mentioned, you and your partner share the same odds for being the source of infertility. While infertility can be devastating to you, it can equally be so for him. Many men take infertility as an affront to their masculinity, and the fact that they cannot father a child bruises their ego. Let us reiterate that mutual support is imperative as you go through the process of trying to find and treat the cause of infertility. In regard to male infertility, the most common causes can be traced to sperm disorders, sexually transmitted diseases, varicocele (hernia of veins next to the testicle), genetic defects, and cystic fibrosis.

Sperm disorders typically involve one of the following two things: the

---

Postcoital means "after intercourse." *Coitus* is another name for intercourse.

production of too few sperm, or adequate production but abnormally shaped sperm. During the initial infertility evaluation, we request that your partner undergo a semen analysis. One of the major problems with an initial fertility evaluation is convincing your partner to join the "cup club."* Many men are reluctant to partake in the clinical procedure of ejaculating into a cup, but it is necessary for evaluation of the sperm.

3. I'm worried that my husband and I are infertile. My friend said that if we drink cough syrup our chances would improve.

Hold on to your hats because evidence actually does support this statement. A little-known study conducted in 1982 showed that the drug guiafenesin could increase the quality of cervical mucus.[1] Guiafenesin is an expectorant used to loosen thickened phlegm in upper respiratory tract infections and make it easier for the body to expel the mucus. It's a common ingredient in over-the-counter cough syrups. The researchers hypothesized that guiafenesin could thin cervical mucus, just like it thins nasal mucus, and make it easier for sperm to travel up the birth canal into the uterus. The authors remained uncertain as to the mechanism of action for the improved fertility, but they assumed that it was similar to guiafenesin's actions on respiratory secretions.

Women participating in the study were given 600 mg of guiafenesin daily in the form of Robitussin cough syrup. They took the guiafenesin from the fifth day of their cycle until they had a temperature rise signifying ovulation. In this solitary study, the authors defined the success rate for treating cervical factor infertility as more than 30 percent of patients becoming pregnant. Patients treated with Robitussin had a success rate of 40 percent. So there was a definite success.

This type of therapy is valid *only* for those couples facing cervical factor infertility in which the main cause of infertility is due to the cervical mucus not allowing the sperm to safely travel to the birth canal. Should you pursue this therapy, here are some points to consider. First, before using guiafenesin as an infertility treatment, we recommend seeking the

---

*This is not a jest by the authors. Many men refer to joining the "cup club" since they have to leave their specimen in a cup.

advice of your personal physician. Guiafenesin is considered pregnancy category C, which means no one really knows if it causes any issues with the fetus, but it is more than likely safe. Second, in the event you do use it, one teaspoon of Robitussin contains 100 mg of guiafenesin, so you would need to take two tablespoons of Robitussin daily for approximately ten days to get a similar amount of guiafenesin as the subjects in the study. Third, when you take guiafenesin you need to drink one cup of water per every teaspoon dose in order to thin the mucus. Finally, Robitussin is often combined with other upper respiratory medications. Robitussin combined with decongestants may actually thicken the cervical mucus, so you would want to avoid that combination.

Interestingly, one of the original researchers followed up on his 1982 guiafenesin study with a 2006 study focusing on the diagnosis and treatment of cervical factor abnormalities.[2] He stated that guiafenesin was the cheapest but least effective therapy. While cough syrup is cheap and may increase your chance of getting pregnant, consult your physician first. He or she may be able to offer you more effective treatments.

Recently, a product hit the market called FertileCM* that claims to increase fertility by supporting the production of "fertile-quality" cervical mucus. This product is a dietary supplement, and to the best of our knowledge there is no solid research backing its claims.

4. We have been trying to get pregnant for six months. My mom says we're infertile and need to see a specialist.

No couple wants to hear the word "infertile." In the medical world we do not consider a couple infertile until they have tried to achieve pregnancy for twelve months. But if you or your husband travel for work and are separated during those times when you're most fertile, you should not consider that time as part of the twelve months. For instance, it is not uncommon for men

---

*This information is from the FertileCM Web site and to the best of our knowledge has not been verified by the FDA. "**FertileCM** integrates several key ingredients that have been shown in clinical studies to safely and naturally promote the production of cervical fluids, support the 'thinning' of mucus, increase hydration of the mucin, as well as promote proper mucus alkalinity. In addition, the same ingredient that supports CM production (L-Arginine as nitric oxide precursor) has also been shown to induce endometrial secretion (creating a healthy uterus lining) during implantation time."

and women in the military to be either deployed or in the field on missions and therefore away from their partner for a period of time.

As a physician in the military for a short time, Shawn had women come to him frustrated that they were not pregnant even though they had been trying for the last year. He was always careful to ask them about the duration of their spouse's deployments over the last year, or, if the patient was a soldier, about their own deployments. An average couple in the United States has an 85 percent chance of becoming pregnant during twelve months of trying. If these same couples extend their efforts to twenty-four months, 95 percent of them become pregnant.

If after six months of normal sexual activity you're not pregnant, try not to be too concerned. If you have just come off of birth control pills or injections, then you may have to wait a few months before your periods are back to normal and routine ovulation begins.

5. Someone told me that eating wild yam will increase my chances of getting pregnant.

Multiple articles in print and on the Web describe the benefits of taking wild yam or wild yam extract in order to increase fertility. In our research for this book, we have yet to locate any articles in medical journals to support the claims of these wild yam fans. It's our personal opinion that the wild yam claims are one of the biggest scams of the decade. One of the reasons we feel this to be a scam is that the companies marketing this product cannot substantiate their claims with any scientific data.

Let's look at the wild yam and explore the wide-ranging claims associated with it.

First things first: the wild yam is not related to the sweet potato. It is the rhizome (or root) of a vine and is believed to contain natural progesterone, the hormone that promotes fertility and pregnancy and menstrual regulation. Thus, wild yam is believed to increase fertility and to alleviate the symptoms of some menstrual irregularities. In reality, however, wild yam contains a compound called diosgenin, not progesterone. Although diosgenin is chemically similar to progesterone, your body cannot utilize this compound, which means that when ingested, diosgenin remains chemically inactive in your body. In labs, diosgenin is chemically converted into natural progesterone, but this chemical conversion cannot be performed by your body. When you see a cream at the store that states it contains wild yam extract, realize that you are putting something on your skin that does absolutely nothing for you hormonally. Your body doesn't know how to use it.

We would love to have an herbal product at our disposal, well studied and proven to help, that we could tell our patients to use in order to assist with their fertility, but the simple truth is that many of these products don't work for most groups of women. We recommend that you look for products backed by sound scientific research. There may be anecdotal evidence in support of a product—your friend might say it worked for her—but there is no way to determine for certain if it was actually the product or other circumstances that led to your friend's pregnancy.

We know many women who will seek the advice of the sales clerk at the local health food store before they ask their healthcare provider's advice, and we wish this could be different. Try to be an informed patient and customer and do your research before you buy into something you read about online or hear about from a friend. There are many physicians who would be willing to open the conversation with you regarding supplements and their proper use. Dealing with infertility can leave you feeling desperate and vulnerable to suggestions that may lead you nowhere or may even be hazardous to your health, not to mention your pocketbook. In certain cases, herbal concoctions may very well be the ticket, but let your physician know what you're doing so that together, you can make the most informed decisions possible.

6. My husband wears tighty whities (tight white briefs with elastic around the waist and leg openings), and I heard he should wear boxers to maximize his sperm count.

If you recall, 40 percent of infertility is caused by male factor infertility, and a majority of these cases are a result of inadequate production of sperm. The above assumption persists because the ambient temperature of the testes can affect the quality and quantity of sperm produced.

If you look at the male anatomy, you will notice that the testicles hang a distance from the body. If your husband is cold, immerses himself in cold water, or chooses to walk around nude on a cold day, then his testicles will pull themselves closer to the body. In contrast, if he takes a hot bath or sits in a hot tub for an extended period time, his testicles will drop as far away from the body as they can in order to cool off. There is a reason for all of this. In order for the testes to make adequate and quality sperm they must be of a temperature that is lower than the body's core temperature of 98.6 degrees. By hanging outside of the body, testicles can adjust in temperature. If they didn't need to do so, they probably would be found inside the pelvic cavity like ovaries. Tight underwear holds the testicles close to the body. If the body's warmth raises the temperature of the testes a couple of degrees, then there is a potential that the sperm count could be diminished.

Does this mean that your partner only needs to don boxer shorts for a few days before you have sex so that his sperm count will rise? It takes about ten weeks for the average male to create new sperm. Thus, wearing boxers for a few days before intercourse probably wouldn't be enough time to increase his sperm count. This could be a problem for some men, who may not want to transition to boxer shorts after years of the old white briefs to which they have become accustomed.

And what about tight pants? He may look hot in a nice tight pair of jeans, but if he has low sperm count, consider ousting them from the wardrobe. Unless he wants to look like Billy Ray Cyrus and grow a mullet, tell him the baggy look is in and find him some looser-fitting jeans or chinos.

However, if a sperm count analysis indicates that all is normal, he's good with the underwear he chooses, and maybe you shouldn't chastise him for his selection of pants.

Just to firm up all the facts, let's say your man likes to bike and, like most serious bikers, he wears tight Lycra pants. There is a possibility that he could have a lower sperm count as a result of wearing these tight-fitting pants. In 2003, OB-GYN News reported that extreme bikers, those who logged more than three thousand miles per year, had lower sperm counts, decreased sperm mobility, and scrotal abnormalities.[3] In this report, bicyclists had an 88 percent rate of scrotal abnormalities while nonbicyclists had only a 26 percent rate of abnormalities. The bikers also had only one-third the sperm count of those who didn't ride bikes. If your partner likes to ride his bike and you are having a problem conceiving, then have his sperm tested and let him know that he might want to take up swimming...

perhaps naked, in a warm pool. It's worth a shot. Seriously, though, a word of caution: If he likes to bike, there is no reason to assume he will have a low sperm count.

7. My sister said we should be having sex at least three times a day if we want to get pregnant.

Three times a day?

What if it took you three or four months to get pregnant?

As you know by now, one of the main components for achieving a pregnancy is for the man to have a normal sperm count. Could too much sex deplete his sperm count to the point where it decreases your chances of getting pregnant? If you abstain from sex until you are most fertile, will your chances of pregnancy improve?

A study done in Israel examined this latter question of whether or not abstinence increased the sperm count in men.[4] Men scheduled for a semen analysis are instructed to abstain from sex for two to seven days prior to the test in order to maximize their sperm count. Research by Dr. E. Levitas showed that while the volume of semen increases when a man abstains for ten to fourteen days, sperm quality actually decreases. Levitas has recommended that men abstain for no more than two days if they want to have good-quality sperm in numbers that should be adequate for pregnancy.

Though we now know that a period of abstinence lasting longer than two days is not recommended, the best time to have intercourse is still around those days when you are ovulating. We suggest that you invest in an inexpensive, over-the-counter ovulation prediction kit available at most pharmacies. Similar to the home pregnancy tests, these ovulation kits are urine based. The stick will turn blue when you experience your lieutinizing hormone (LH) surge—the release of LH that signals the ovary to eject an egg (ovulate). When the line on the ovulation stick turns blue, you should be ovulating within the next twenty-four hours. If you start having sex at that point and do so for the next two to three days, you should have your bases covered. Some people call this "sex on demand" because, when the stick turns blue, you can demand that your man pay attention to you. He may fuss a bit, saying things like "he is not your servant," but he'll get over it, and when the baby is two or three years old, he'll look back and wish he could be there again. We say this from personal experiences, one of which Shawn would like to share.

> Years ago when my wife and I made a house-hunting trip to Tucson, she was taking Clomid, a fertility drug that stimulates ovarian egg production. Women who are on this medication and use ovulation urine tests know exactly when they ovulate. When the stick turns blue, it's time to "get it on."
>
> One day, while dealing with the stress of searching for a home, we got entrenched in a bitter argument. Suddenly, by cosmic chance, she remembered it was day fourteen of her cycle—the day she'd likely release an egg. Immediately, her demeanor shifted to that of the hunter—and I, her desired sexual prey, was in her sights.
>
> Still emotionally involved in our argument, I wasn't in the mood to have sex right then. I protested. How could I give up the fruit of my loins just because she said it was time? How could a sexual encounter even be scheduled like a stuffy luncheon? And I certainly couldn't be "had" because the date of her cycle said so. Who am I? Sing-Sing, the giant almost-extinct panda? No, I'm a man, a man with needs beyond the physical and I have to be ready too.
>
> Well, I ended up giving in. Now, we have an orange-headed boy who loves Buddha. (I'm not certain if his love for Buddha was borne of the bondage of my oppression, but I'd like to think so.) Several years, four children, and two busy medical careers later, I sometimes wish my wife would look at me that way again.

8. The reason you are not getting pregnant is that your partner masturbates.

If your partner is masturbating so many times a day that it interferes with normal daily activities, including your relationship, then you—and he— may have a problem. Up to 95 percent of men claim that they masturbate at least once a day. In this case, his sperm count will not decrease significantly unless you are having sex within a few hours after he ejaculates. Masturbation with ejaculation cleans out his pipes and makes room for new sperm. As long as you've had his sperm count checked and everything is normal, then his masturbating is not something to fret over.

In our society masturbation has its own mythology. In religious circles, it often carries a negative connotation. Masturbation comes from the Latin word *masturbare*, the roots of which are *manus* (hand) and *stuprare* (defile); if you masturbate, you are defiling with the hand. For centuries, various religions have taught that masturbation is a sin, yet the medical community has discovered no evidence that masturbation is either physically or mentally harmful. So let's do a little debunking. The following myths may seem funny in this day and age, but it was only thirty to fifty years ago that they were considered truths.

- Masturbation causes hairy palms. Considering that about 95 percent of men and 65 percent of women masturbate and no one is demanding laser treatments for hairy palms, it's easy to prove this statement is false.
- Masturbation makes you go blind. Can you imagine?
- Masturbation makes you sterile. The reality is that many experts think that masturbation can add to a healthy sex life and a sexually healthy individual.
- Masturbation will make your penis shrink, cause acne, give you a sexually transmitted disease, and could potentially cause you to become sexually perverted. This sounds like the basis of some sex education program in the 1950s. All false.

9. Pregnancy will happen if you just relax.

Who hasn't heard the story of the couple that has tried to get pregnant for years? She peed on so many pregnancy and ovulation test sticks that she sees them in her dreams. Shots in the butt and blood tests with pelvic ultrasounds became as routine as having toast for breakfast. She knows more about the menstrual cycle and hormones than most ob-gyn residents, and he has become more proficient at injections than the nurse administering vaccines at the local pediatric clinic. They have spent thousands of dollars on one singular mission: getting pregnant. They want a baby badly, but they haven't been able to have one. After months and even years of trying, they finally give up. The next month, voilà. They're pregnant, and why are they pregnant? Everyone thinks it's because they finally stopped trying so hard and just relaxed.

Could it be that couples enduring the stressors of infertility can propagate their problems with their own stress? This particular type of stress
and its resulting disease process has a name—mindset-infertility—and
there are psychologists who specialize in treating it. Mindset-infertility is
based on animal studies that show that when certain species experience
stress, their reproductive functions become stressed. Although such studies
have not been done with humans, it makes sense to extrapolate the findings
to our species, particularly since we have scientifically determined that
stress affects our physicality. Why would our reproductive organs be
exempt from the damaging affects of stress?

Take a deep breath and relax. You might be attempting to control a
host of things if you have infertility issues. Try to control those things that
you yourself CAN control, like checking for ovulation and getting decent
nutrition, sleep, and exercise. Focus on taking care of yourself and let the
other things fall into place.

10. I already have one child, so I will have no problem conceiving a second child.

Before you jump to this conclusion, you need to answer a few questions.
Are you with the same partner with whom you had the first child? If you
have changed partners, does your new partner have any infertility issues
such as a low sperm count? Has your medical or surgical history changed
since you were last pregnant? The onset of a disease like endometriosis or
scarring from surgery could affect your ability to get pregnant. Some sexually transmitted diseases like chlamydia and gonorrhea can contribute to
tubal factor infertility by causing an inflammation of the tubes. If you have
developed pelvic pain and could possibly have endometriosis, then there is
a risk that you could also have tubal factor infertility from damage to the
fallopian tubes. Are you close to the same age as when you first conceived?
Age can play a factor in the success rates of your pregnancy attempts. As
you age, it's harder to conceive. If you had your first child fifteen years ago
when you were twenty-five years old and now you are trying to conceive
at age forty, you can still get pregnant. Just know that it may take more tries
than it did the first time around. (We'll delve further into this topic in the
next chapter.)

Suffice it to say, if all of your medical and surgical history is unchanged, and all remains the same between you and your partner, and he hasn't started wearing snug spandex pants to work, then the above assumption is not a myth. Your chances of getting pregnant again are likely the same as they were before.

11. Infertility is only a problem for older women.

A patient called the office, irate because of a medical coding issue that revolved around her age. When we received the phone message from one of the office billing staff, we wondered what on earth the patient could be upset about, as we had routinely referred her to a high-risk specialist (maternal fetal medicine). She was thirty-eight years old and pregnant with her second child. We wanted her to take advantage of genetic counseling, which entails meeting with a high-risk obstetrical physician and a genetic counselor. These doctors advise patients of the risks based on their age and the chances of them having an infant with a chromosomal abnormality. The information is then used to guide the patient through the decision of whether or not to have a genetic amniocentesis, a process in which some of the fluid surrounding the baby is withdrawn through a needle and sent to a lab for a chromosomal analysis. The baby's skin cells are removed from the fluid and tested for chromosomal issues.

My patient was upset because she had received her bill from the specialist's office and they had used a bothersome ICD-9 code for the visit. An ICD-9 code is a set of numbers sent to the insurance company to alert them as to why the patient had the visit. In this patient's case, they used the code V23.82.

"Do you know what a V23.82 is?" she asked. "It stands for Elderly Multigravida! Elderly?" she questioned, aghast.

A multigravida refers to a woman who has been pregnant more than once, but we think she was more upset with the word *elderly*, and wouldn't you be, too? Someone at Medicare must have thought it was a good idea to label women over the age of thirty-five as elderly. It was a bad idea. Fortunately, that code has been changed, and now we use the politically correct term *advanced maternal age* (AMA) to refer to women over the age of thirty-five.

In the context of fertility, however, thirty-five is not a magical number. There is really only one reason the definition of AMA is cut off at thirty-five. It's all about chromosomes. The risk of a woman of thirty-five having a chromosomally abnormal infant is 1 in 200. The test to determine this, an amniocentesis, discussed above, carries the risk of miscarriage of 1 in 200. Therefore, the risk of the procedure is the same as the risk of the possible diagnosis, so the test can be indicated at that point. Also, the reality is that a woman's fertility does start decreasing around age thirty, and that's all about the eggs and the chromosomes within them. A woman is born with all the eggs she will ever have. These eggs "die off," so to speak, every day of her life. So, when the woman is thirty-five, these eggs have been around for thirty-five years and have been exposed to ambient radiation and all that the environment has to offer. Subsequently they can become damaged and less healthy and thereby less fertile. At the age of thirty-five there is a steep drop, and around age thirty-eight there is another steep decline.

Is infertility a problem for "older" women? Not necessarily. You don't know until you try. We were fortunate to have two children later in life when Katie was thirty-six and then thirty-nine. The facts show that any woman under the age of thirty has about a 20 percent chance of becoming pregnant each month. A woman over the age of forty has about a 5 percent chance monthly. Also, the fertility rate, which is the amount of births per thousand women with the potential to become pregnant, drops significantly from age thirty-five to forty-five, from 400 per 1,000 exposed women, to 100 per 1,000 women exposed.[5]

12. Infertility drugs increase your chances of twins and triplets.

You've got it. This is no myth.

One of the first line of drugs used in infertility treatments is Clomid,* or clomiphene citrate. Because about 25 percent of female factor infertility involves ovulatory issues, Clomid is a relatively common medication.

---

*This medication is used to treat infertility in women. It works by stimulating an increase in the amount of hormones that support the growth and release of a mature egg (ovulation). This medication is not recommended for women whose ovaries no longer make eggs properly (primary pituitary or ovarian failure).

Chances are either you or someone you know has taken this medication. Clomid is prescribed to help restore normal ovulation in women with irregular or absent ovulatory periods. Once ovulation becomes regular, the drug is continued through six menstrual cycles. Studies show that its benefits decrease substantially after six cycles. Forty to forty-five percent of patients on Clomid will achieve pregnancy within the first six months of use.[6] However, Clomid does increase the chance of multiple births. If you're on Clomid, you have an approximately 10 percent chance of having twins and less than a 1 percent chance of having triplets.

One popular myth regarding medications is that if a little works, more must work better. In the case of Clomid, if a little fixes your ovulatory problems, then more should increase ovulation, right? Wrong. Increasing the dose of Clomid without supervision can lead to a thickening of the cervical mucus and thus decrease your fertility. Remember, if the sperm can't get into the uterus, you can't get pregnant.

Another set of fertility medications that can increase the rates of multiple births are the human gonadotropins (Pergonal, Metrodin, Humagon). To describe how these drugs interact with the body and the painstaking way they are used would require another book. For our purposes, let's focus on the risk of multiple births that accompanies these types of medications. Approximately one-fourth of the patients using human gonadotropins will have twins; 2 to 3 percent will have triplets, and one in one hundred pregnancies will have four or more babies. These medications are expensive at $2,000 per cycle, but they definitely offer more bang for the buck to couples suffering from ovulation irregularities.

Medicine has advanced far in its ability to treat infertility. Myths continue to pervade, however. As with any medical issue, we encourage you to consult your personal physician or healthcare provider to learn how best to proceed. The odds are that you will get pregnant at some point. When this happens, you will move into a new world replete with its own set of myths. We would like to introduce you to some of the myths, moods, and mothers of that world. We'll begin by exploring the myths associated with early pregnancy, that time when physical and emotional changes begin, including an increase in appetite.

Notes

1. H. J. Check and H. G. Adelson, "Improvement of Cervical Factor with Guiafenesin," *Fertility and Sterility* 37, no. 5 (1982): 706.

2. H. J. Check, "Diagnosis and Treatment of Cervical Mucus Abnormalities," *Clinical and Experimental Obstetrics & Gynecology* 33, no. 3 (2006): 140.

3. http://findarticles.com/p/articles/mi_m0CYD/is_3_38/ai_97850490 (accessed April 11, 2009).

4. E. Levitas et al., "Relationship between the Duration of Sexual Abstinence and Semen Quality: Analysis of 9,489 Semen Samples," *Fertility and Sterility* 83, no. 6 (2005): 1680.

5. Linda Heffner, "Advanced Maternal Age—How Old Is Too Old?" *New England Journal of Medicine* 351, no. 19 (2004): 1927.

6. http://www.asrm.org/Patients/patientbooklets/ovulation_drugs.pdf (accessed April 18, 2009).

Chapter Three

Conception Myths
The Voodoo against You

Y ou want to have a baby. You long to hear the little pitter-pat of feet on the tile floor, and hearing those words "mama" and "dada" is your most sought-after goal. Prior to getting pregnant, many of our patients ask a plethora of questions. What sexual positions are best for conceiving? When is the best time in my menstrual cycle to become pregnant? Of course, not every patient is ready to have a baby. Those who aren't are asking questions like "When during my cycle do I particularly avoid having sex?" and "Do I still need birth control if I've never had an orgasm?" Perhaps you've heard more than one answer for each of these questions from your girlfriends, your great-aunt, or the woman next to you on the subway. That's because myths still mingle with facts. Whether you want to conceive a child or want to avoid conception, you need to distill fact from fiction. So here we go.

1. I can't become pregnant the first time I have sex.

This is one of the primary conception myths floating around out there, especially among teens and tweens. Peer pressure to have sex and lack of sexual education might be keeping this myth alive. One friend passes the misinformation on to another who passes it on to another. So let's set the record straight, particularly for all our younger readers. (We have a fifteen-year-old daughter and we hope she is reading this section.) If you are of reproductive age, which means you have started your period—and in this country that can be as early as age nine—then anytime you have unprotected sex, you can become pregnant. Even the first time you have sex, there is a chance of getting pregnant. We ask you, regardless of age or parental status, to keep this information alive and circulating: If you have started your period, then it is possible for you to get pregnant anytime you have unprotected sex. Hillary's story exemplifies how this myth can dramatically change the course of one's life.

Hillary, a thirteen-year-old with light auburn hair, smooth-as-silk, freckly skin, and a sweet disposition, came to our clinic with complaints of lower abdominal pains. Her mother drove her and was concerned that her daughter might have a urinary tract infection. Her urine specimen tested normal, so I interviewed Hillary a bit more, asking if her periods were painful or irregular since she started having them six months ago. She said that she had four periods, then missed the last two months. This pattern can be normal in a young girl who has just started her menses. I also asked her if she was sexually active, and she shyly said no. Her mother laughed nervously, and I could tell that she was somewhat put off by my question. I apologized for asking and explained that we see girls Hillary's age with positive pregnancy tests. Hillary then asked if she could go on birth control pills to help her periods become more regular and less painful, two things the pills can do besides preventing pregnancy. I spent the next few minutes going over the specifics of oral contraceptives and how to use them. If you miss one pill then take two the next day. If you miss two pills, then take two pills the next two days and if you miss three pills, use condoms until you start your next period. I walked out of the room and out of habit, asked my medical assistant to run a urine pregnancy test, a protocol when starting someone on medications.

My assistant showed me the pregnancy test before I returned to the room. The line on it had turned blue. At age thirteen, Hillary was pregnant. She was going to be a fourteen-year-old mother.

Walking back into that room was one of the harder things I've done. I'm not saying that other patient situations haven't been difficult, but I will never forget the surprise, then the devastation I saw on the faces of mother and daughter when I relayed the news.

Hillary later explained that one of her older male friends had said that she didn't need to worry about pregnancy if it was her first time having sex. He had read this in a magazine and managed to convince her that having unprotected sex was safe. She fell prey to the myth. Now she and her mother had to deal with many difficult decisions. Hillary chose to have the baby, and she and her daughter lived with her parents while she continued going to school. A very motivated young woman with a wonderful future ahead of her, she recently graduated from high school. She did admit that being pregnant in middle school and high school caused her to lose most of her friends. It proved to be a very challenging and trying time. Hillary now volunteers at a local teen pregnancy program and mentors other young women who are pregnant.

2. Today is the fourteenth day of my period, so I won't get pregnant.

In order to understand this myth, we need to look at some basics of the menstrual cycle. There are two distinct phases. The first half of the cycle is called the *proliferative phase*, and the second half is called the *secretory phase*. The proliferative phase begins right after menstrual bleeding stops and continues until ovulation. As you know, ovulation occurs when an egg is released from the ovary. Since no egg is released and available for fertilization during the proliferative phase, you cannot become pregnant during this time. This is the opposite of the speculative stage, which begins at ovulation and continues until you start bleeding. During the speculative stage, you *can* become pregnant.

Although you can't get pregnant during the proliferative phase, the problem with relying on this phase as birth control is that its length varies slightly from cycle to cycle. If you have a thirty-five-day cycle, meaning thirty-five days from the first day of a period until the first day of the next period, you might ovulate on or around the twenty-first day, but not necessarily exactly on the twenty-first day of each cycle. Similarly, a woman who has a twenty-four-day cycle might ovulate on or around the tenth day of her cycle, but not necessarily on the tenth day. Another variable that comes into play is the life span of the sperm and the egg. Both live between twenty-four and forty-eight hours. Let's say you have a twenty-four-day cycle and you assume you ovulate on day fourteen. If you have intercourse on day twelve, you might assume you're in the safety zone and won't get pregnant. The sperm, however, might live for forty-eight hours, in which case they are alive and swimming on the day you ovulate. If a sperm hooks up with the egg released by your ovary on day fourteen, touchdown! You will find yourself pregnant.

Now, some women choose the type of natural birth control that requires monitoring basal body temperature and cervical mucus consistency and keeping meticulous records. In a normal cycle there is a progesterone surge around twenty-four hours following ovulation, and this progesterone surge causes a slight body temperature increase. Because this increase is subtle and rarely exceeds one degree, you must use a basal body thermometer (BBT) that is graded for this measurement. During ovulation, cervical mucus also becomes thicker, and there is a way of determining and charting this using systems like the Creighton Model Fertility Care (CrMS).* Women who use the CrMS can quote an efficacy rate of 99.5 percent in the first year.[1] Yet, even effective birth control will be ineffective if not used correctly, and there is certainly great potential for human error here.

> Anne was a motivated, educated thirty-two-year-old mother of three who wanted to avoid any possible side effects of birth control pills. Oral contraceptives ("the pill") that use synthetic estrogens, and injections that utilize synthetic progesterone may cause mild side effects like nausea, weight gain, mood changes, and lighter periods. Less common are more serious side effects like abdominal pain, chest pain, headaches, eye problems, and swelling or aches in the legs and thighs. She decided to follow a natural birth control plan that included monitoring her estrogen and progesterone levels along with checking basal body temperatures and cervical mucus. She had been using the method for about three months and noticed that she had missed her period. A home pregnancy test came out positive.
>
> When she came in for her initial OB visit we started talking about the possible way she became pregnant. She had followed instructions to the letter.
>
> "Was there anything about the data you were collecting that just didn't seem right?" I asked.

---

*For more information on this method of natural birth control, please go to http://www .creightonmodel.com.

She thought for a minute and said, "Well, my body temperatures were always flat. They never seemed to show the temperature spike indicating ovulation. I just thought I was weird and didn't have that spike."

She had brought the temperature charts, and they indeed looked flat. Anne said she did use a basal body thermometer, so I asked her how she was taking her temperature. She said that every morning before she got out of bed, she placed the thermometer in her vagina, waited a few minutes, and then read the temperature and recorded it.

"I think I see the problem," I said.

"What?"

"It's an oral thermometer."

3. I was told that certain sexual positions are better than others for conceiving.

Is there really a sexual position that can increase chances of conception? Although no definitive scientific studies answer this question, theories abound. Couples have been having sex in the "man-on-top" missionary position for centuries, and this seems to work well for most couples. It's a position that maximizes the amount of sperm deposited on the cervix and increases the amount of time it stays there. If you can stay lying down comfortably after intercourse, this will help keep your partner's semen in your vagina and potentially increase the return on your investment, because his sperm has a greater chance of making it into the birth canal. You may want to avoid positions where gravity is not working in your favor, such as the "woman-on-top" positions. If you straddle your partner, for instance, there is a greater chance that his semen will flow away from your cervix and even run out of you. Enough said.

4. I have never had an orgasm, and my friend said that my boyfriend and I have to orgasm together in order for me to get pregnant. Do I still need birth control?

While it's generally true male orgasm is generally essential for you to become pregnant, a small possibility exists that even if he does *not* have an

orgasm, you could still become pregnant. There are even less-likely incidences when the male partner does not ejaculate, but sperm from the vis-
cous material that precedes the semen can actually fertilize an egg. So the
answer to this question is YES! You *do* still need birth control. The whole
truth is that neither you nor your partner need to have an orgasm for you
to get pregnant. This myth may be perpetuated by the fact that female
orgasm causes involuntary uterine contractions and that these contractions
propel the sperm up into the fallopian tubes.

One Web site explains the connection between orgasm and conception
as follows:

- Orgasm helps to increase the chances of conception.
- Orgasm increases the blood flow to the reproductive organs, helping
  them to function better.
- Orgasm also helps the cervix to "suck" up sperm in the vagina, thus
  helping the sperm to reach the awaiting egg.[2]

A study done in 2006 found that women who fake orgasms have the
same conception rate as women who experience real orgasms.[3] What an
interesting study to design and conduct, no doubt. Scientists are intrigued
by female orgasm, since it seems to be unnecessary for conception, unlike
the male orgasm, which usually is necessary. Is the female orgasm a lost
piece of evolution like the appendix or is it possibly a vestige that has
stayed with us for the sole purpose of fun and pleasure? Some scientists
believe that the female orgasm has merely tagged along the evolutionary
scale with the male orgasm.[4] They have likened the female orgasm to male
nipples in the sense that while female nipples serve a purpose, male nipples are a tagalong from female evolution. Our counterpoint question to
these scientists is this: would women truly want to have sex if there were
no feeling or potential reward of orgasm? Would women only want to have
sex to propagate the species? Many women would still want to have intercourse, because they would want to have babies. But for women who enjoy
orgasm, it just wouldn't be the same.

5. I am thirty-five years old and want to start a family. I heard my chances of getting pregnant are less than when I was twenty.

In general, women experience decreased pregnancy rates as they age. In 2006, National Vital Statistics Reports collected the following data, which were reported by the Centers for Disease Control and Prevention in 2007.[5] Note that these rates are for the populations as a whole and do not focus only on women seeking to become pregnant.

- Between 2005 and 2006, the general fertility rate increased by 3 percent to 68.5 births per 1,000 women aged 15 to 44. This increase was the largest on record since 1991.
- Teenagers aged 15 to 19 had a birthrate of 41.9 births per 1,000 women.
- Women aged 20 to 24 had a birthrate of 105.9 per 1,000.
- Women aged 25 to 29 had a birthrate of 116.8 per 1,000.
- Women aged 30 to 34 had a birthrate of 97.7 per 1,000.
- Women aged 35 to 39 had a birthrate of 47.3 per 1,000, an increase of 3 percent from 2005.
- Women aged 40 to 44 had a birthrate of 9.4 per 1,000, an increase of 3 percent from 2005.
- Women aged 45 to 49 had a birthrate of 0.9 per 1,000, a 1 percent increase from 2005.

As you can see, a woman hits her peak birthrate from ages 25 to 29, wherein begins a steady and rapid decline. Your chances of getting pregnant at age 35 are less than half of what they were from ages 20 to 24. Your chances of getting pregnant at the age of 45 are about 1,000 times lower than from ages 20 to 24. While you might argue that you have more wisdom and experience to be a mother in your later years, nature doesn't appear to agree. You could argue, though, that birthrates are lower in older women because not as many are attempting to get pregnant and more have undergone permanent sterilization.

6. I'm presently breastfeeding so I can't get pregnant.

The answer is yes, and the answer is no.

Overall, breastfeeding is a decent form of birth control and is officially called the Lactational Amenorrhea Method (LAM).* As with other birth control methods, LAM has to be used correctly in order to be effective. The criteria for using LAM is as follows:

- Your baby must be under six months old.
- Your baby is almost exclusively breastfed. This means you aren't supplementing with formula. Some experts say that the baby should not be ingesting more than two mouthfuls per day of water or other foods.
- Your baby is feeding regularly during the day and night. The baby should go no more than four hours between breastfeeding during the day and no more than six hours between breastfeeding during the night.
- Your menstrual periods have not yet resumed.

If these guidelines are followed to a T, LAM has a pregnancy rate of between one to two pregnancies per one hundred women. This is slightly worse than the pill, which reports pregnancy rates of 0.3 per one hundred women. LAM is a better form of birth control than condoms or diaphragms. Of course, you can get pregnant if you are breastfeeding, since nothing short of a hysterectomy is 100 percent effective, but used properly, LAM is a fine form of birth control. It is also true that some women rely on breastfeeding not just for nutrition but to comfort their infants. These women will have a higher incidence of infertility for the first three to six months postpartum than those women whose children rely on pacifiers and drinks like water or juice for comfort. It has also been reported that women using LAM had improved fetal and maternal health.

In order to maintain infertility while breastfeeding, make sure you feed your baby the same amount of breast milk and breastfeed for the same length of time every day. Women who return to work or introduce solid

---

*La Leche League International is a wonderful resource for anything regarding breastfeeding. They have information regarding LAM on their Web site at http://www.LLLI.org.

foods into their baby's diet may find that they have returned to ovulating. Before beginning work or expanding your baby's diet, you may to want to add another form of birth control.

If you are interested in learning more about LAM as a form of birth control, please visit the Web site listed in the notes section at the end of this chpater[6] or call your local La Leche League office for information. If you go to your provider with the desire to breastfeed solely as a form of birth control, please bring your information to your postpartum visit. Many obstetricians and gynecologists don't have a good grasp on the intricacies of breastfeeding and what mothers are being taught before they leave the hospital. This is a good time to educate your doctor after you have educated yourself. We believe that most healthcare providers would be more than happy to explore this method with you and help you make it work to the best of their ability, as long as they feel you are informed of the strengths and weaknesses of whichever method you choose.

7. I won't get pregnant because my partner "pulls out" before he ejaculates.

Coitus interruptus, or "pulling out," is fairly common among teenagers who are either afraid to seek medical attention for birth control, can't afford to, or don't want to buy condoms. They don't want to alert their parents that they are sexually active, and many of them pay the price for this discretion after they have a positive pregnancy test. As with many other forms of birth control, withdrawal does not prevent sexually transmitted diseases either.

Even when this method is used consistently and correctly, studies show a failure rate of 15 to 28 percent.[7] This failure could be attributable to a fluid called Cowper's fluid, which is emitted from the penis prior to ejaculation. This pre-ejaculate fluid can carry sperm that could make their way into the uterus and fallopian tubes. A greater risk, however, occurs if your male partner has recently ejaculated and the sperm remains inside the urethra of the penis when you have intercourse. The sperm in his urethra can be swept into the Cowper's fluid and deposited in the vagina.

A final note on coitus interruptus: you are counting on your partner to stop short of orgasm and pull his penis out of you. This requires a partner who is on the same page as you in the sense that he is able to think at the moment of truth and not continue in the heat of the moment. This method is especially problematic if you have no idea when he is getting close to ejaculation.

8. I was told if I have sex during my period then I won't get pregnant.

When you start your period each month, there is no ovulated egg in your fallopian tubes. The reason you begin bleeding is because ovulation occurred but a sperm did not fertilize your egg, so no pregnancy was implanted in the uterus. The thickened endometrial lining of the uterus is now in the process of sloughing. Theoretically, you can't get pregnant during this sloughing (bleeding), again because there is no egg hanging around waiting to meet a sperm. But never say never, because in rare instances, having sex during your period might result in a pregnancy. Furthermore, there are other reasons to be bleeding, besides a period. Some women have bleeding during ovulation. Granted, it is usually not as significant a bleed as a menstrual period, but it certainly is not a sure thing.

The National Institutes of Health (NIH) conducted a study in 2005 that found that women could be fertile as early as four days from the start of their menstrual flow; in this study 17 percent of women were fertile by day seven. Your fertile time lasts about one week per month, and after you ovulate your egg is alive for twenty-four to forty-eight hours. As discussed earlier, there are times in a woman's life, such as perimenopause or in teenage years when the menstrual cycle may be irregular, that make it difficult to ascertain whether bleeding is a true menstrual flow or something called dysfunctional uterine bleeding, which means abnormal bleeding due to irregular ovulation.

Take, for example, a woman who has a disorder like polycystic ovarian disease, in which she makes many eggs but none of them ovulates (release of an egg from the ovary). Consequently, she may not experience menses for six months at a time. Bleeding then may occur for two different reasons. She may have bleeding because she does indeed ovulate and menstrual bleeding follows about fourteen days later. She may also have bleeding because the lining of her uterus is so thickened by the continuous effects of estrogen that she sheds excess lining, which is not technically a true period. This second situation indicates a time when the woman could become pregnant. If you're one of those women with irregular menses, please be aware that it will be extremely difficult for you to know when you are ovulating.

⟡

We have looked at a few of the conception myths that could be reasons for some pregnancies. If you are ever in doubt of a situation in which you might become pregnant, stop and place a call to your physician, or, better yet, just assume that you are always fertile; the best offense is a good defense. This is true for women in the perimenopausal years as well.

> Janet was a forty-three-year-old woman who came to the office for an annual exam. While interviewing her and reviewing her past medical history, I noticed that she wasn't on any form of birth control. She claimed that her last doctor told her that she "could never" get pregnant because she had a disorder called endometriosis. Endometriosis is a process in which the lining of the uterus can become implanted inside the abdomen or pelvis, causing inflammation that can decrease pregnancy rates. Severe cases of endometriosis can cause infertility by blocking or interfering with tubal function. I had a lengthy discussion with her regarding the fact that I never say "always" or "never" in my practice, because I have witnessed the unexpected too many times. She laughed and said that she would call me if she got pregnant. About eight months later, I opened the door to one of my exam rooms and there sat a calm Janet and her bewildered husband.
>
> "Here I am," she said.
>
> "What's going on?" I asked.
>
> "Remember how I told you I would call you if I ever got pregnant? Well, I thought I would just come in instead."
>
> She eventually went on and delivered her baby nine months later without complications, and this time around she asked me to tie her tubes.

Notes

1. http://www.creightonmodel.com/effectiveness.htm (accessed January 2, 2009).

2. http://sexeducation.lifetips.com/cat/60941/orgasms/index.html#tip-94958 (accessed January 2, 2009).

3. M. Zuk, "The Case of the Female Orgasm," *Perspectives in Biology and Medicine* 49, no. 2 (2006): 294.

4. D. Symons, *The Evolution of Human Sexuality* (New York: Oxford University Press, 1979).

5. http://www.cdc.gov/nchs/data/nvsr/nvsr56/nvsr56_07.pdf (accessed January 10, 2009).

6. http://www.llli.org/ba/Aug93.html (accessed January 10, 2009).

7. J. Kippley and S. Kippley, *The Art of Natural Family Planning*, 4th ed. (Cincinnati: Couple to Couple League, 1996).

Section Three
Early Pregnancy and Mood Myths

Chapter Four

Dietary Myths
What's Eating You?

The "seed" has been planted, so to speak, and now you are officially pregnant. You have given your body over to another life for the next nine months. By the time you can see that fetus on an ultrasound, it's about the size of a sunflower seed or a grain of rice. And that little grain of rice has a heartbeat that you can see and hear. The moment of seeing and hearing your baby's heartbeat is only one morsel in a feast of miraculous maternal moments awaiting you. Your purpose now is to provide a healthy vessel in which your baby can grow and thrive. Your health is your baby's health. This is your very first chance to provide your baby with an optimal start to life, and it's all up to you. The father doesn't have anything to do with this one. It's all yours.

How do you do it? How do you maintain your best possible health for this precious little grain of rice? Nutrition, nutrition, nutrition. Everything you put in your mouth has the potential to affect this baby, and yet most of what you put in your mouth doesn't even reach it. Let me explain. For the most part, the food you eat is converted to calories and energy to assist your body's newly increased metabolism. To put it simply, your body needs energy to sustain pregnancy. Here's a quick and easy two-sentence lesson on the human digestive tract. The food you eat is digested in your gastrointestinal tract. The nutrients from that food are then absorbed into your bloodstream, where some filter through to the placenta and into the baby's bloodstream. That's how *some* of what you eat gets to the baby. Note the operative word "some." Not everything you eat makes it to the baby.

The above lesson gives you the basis to understand the many dietary myths you will encounter during this time of growth. It might also help you grow the baby and not grow you, if you know what I mean.

1. My grandmother says I have to eat more because I am eating for two.

Although this myth, like any, should be taken with a grain of salt, it contains an element of truth. Yes, you are eating for two, but the second one you're eating for will rarely exceed ten pounds at the end of his or her stay. So you're eating for a miniature human who ranges in size from a grain of rice to a small watermelon. Thus, this statement rings true as long as you don't interpret it to mean that you should eat double the food.

How much do you need to eat? Let's talk quantity. We'll get to quality a bit later. A woman who is an average weight for her height requires about 250 extra calories a day during pregnancy. If you are not a calorie counter, these calories equate to an extra peanut butter and jelly sandwich a day. Another example would be precisely two and a half 100-calorie snack bags of Oreo cookies or Goldfish crackers a day. Those are certainly not quality choices, but, as I said, we'll get to that topic later.

But what if you are not an average-sized person? What if you are very small or very large, or just thin or overweight? There is a formula we use in medicine called a Body Mass Index, or BMI. This formula takes into account your height and weight and gives you a number. There is a range of these numbers that is universally accepted as healthy. A BMI of 18.5 to 24.9 is considered normal. The formula is:

$$BMI = weight\ in\ kilograms/height\ in\ meters$$

You are underweight if you have a BMI of less than 18.5, and you are overweight if you have a BMI of 25 to 29.9. You are obese if you are 30 or over.

The BMI helps establish "average" or healthy weights. If you're either underweight or overweight, the amount of extra calories you need to consume in order to maintain your pregnancy will depend on how many calories you already consume. If you are overweight, it stands to reason that you are already consuming more calories than an "average" person. So when figuring out how many calories you need to consume, you need to use another formula called the basal metabolic rate, or BMR. The formula is as follows:

$$\text{BMR} = 655 + (4.35 \times \text{weight in pounds}) + (4.7 \times \text{height in inches}) - (4.7 \times \text{age in years})$$

The above formula is then multiplied by 1.2 for a person who does little or no activity at all, 1.375 for someone who exercises lightly one to three times a week, 1.55 for moderate exercise three to five times a week, and 1.725 for heavy exercise six to seven times a week. So now add 250 calories to the BMR total and, voilà, here is, roughly, the amount of calories you should be consuming to maintain a healthy baby and a healthy you. If you aren't a numbers person, you can find many online calculators for the BMI and BMR formulas that do the math for you.

These are precise formulas meant to be used to calculate an approximate goal, not to be used strictly for a diet of calorie counting during pregnancy. They are meant to be a guideline, tools for self-awareness and methods for checking to ensure that you're not really eating for two adult-sized people.

2. Pregnant women crave pickles and ice cream.

Do pregnant women really crave this infamous combo, the one referenced on sitcoms and about as cliché as the phrase "eating for two"? I can honestly say that I have never had a patient tell me she craved those particular items, at least not at the same time. Many women treat themselves to ice cream frequently. If you feel the need to "treat" yourself, you may be feeling restricted or deprived in some way. You might be experiencing deprivation from things you are used to consuming as a daily habit, things you have come to depend on, such as sodas or coffee. Now all of a sudden, on the day that pregnancy test turns positive, you are expected to give those things up without a fight, without any difficulty at all. Or maybe you are feeling especially tired or nauseous, or bloated, or you're having a hard time breathing or sleeping comfortably. The list could go on and on since everyone experiences pregnancy differently. Maybe you're not feeling restricted in any way but just want an excuse to eat ice cream. Either way, we don't really think women crave ice cream. They just want to enjoy the pleasure it offers.

About the pickles... we just can't say. We have not had anyone tell us of a craving for them. If one did, we might consider the type of pickle she wanted. Is it sweet, sour, or dill? There does seem to be a common craving that includes a citrus, sour, sweet combination, or a sweet and salty combination. We see this commonly. Katie had a constant craving for lemonade when she was pregnant. Was her body deficient in vitamin C? Or did it just sound good because it might settle her stomach because of nausea or get rid of the metallic taste in her mouth that began shortly after the nausea started?

One Friday night my husband and I went out to a Mexican food restaurant. It was very crowded, so rather than wait with the vibrating pager to tell us when our table might be ready, we opted to sit at the bar where we could gorge on chips and salsa and have no room for the entrees we would eat anyway. So my husband, not pregnant, ordered a margarita. I, pregnant, ordered a virgin margarita. (For those of you who might not know, "virgin" is another way of saying "without alcohol" in cocktail lingo.) I couldn't get enough of that lemony sour taste. I took one sip and turned to my husband and said, "This is the BEST virgin margarita I have ever had!" And come to think of it, I don't think I had ever really had a virgin margarita. But anyway, I was only eight weeks pregnant, and I thought to myself, I won't even miss that alcohol taste at all. These are really tasty. After a few more sips, I began to feel a slight warmth down my throat, and became a little suspicious that there might be a little more to my drink. I asked my husband to take a sip, and he agreed it was quite tasty. I became concerned at this point that there was a slight chance I might be drinking tequila. So I got the bartender's attention and told him how good the virgin margarita was. I then asked, "There isn't any alcohol in this, is there?" To which he laughed and replied, "You bet there is... at least two shots." He obviously didn't understand my use of the word "virgin." Perhaps it was the twenty-five-year-age difference between us.

Anyway, no more virgin margaritas for me. It didn't stop me from continuing to drink lemonade, though, and eating lemon bars and sour patch candies, and anything sweet and sour that I could get my hands on. And yes, I gained more weight than I should have.

3. Food cravings mean I have a nutritional deficiency.

What exactly is a craving? Is it an evolutionary mechanism of the human body divinely designed to provide guidance for nutrition that will sustain the species? Cravings have been studied at length, and yet no definitive answers to these questions exist. Personally, we tend to think they are more behavior related rather than mediated by actual nutritional need.

There is one condition, though, that definitely connects a nutritional deficiency to a craving. It is called pica. This is a syndrome that results from iron deficiency anemia. Iron deficiency anemia occurs when red blood cells lack sufficient hemoglobin, which is responsible for carrying oxygen throughout the body. While this type of anemia is very common in pregnancy, pica occurs only in a very small percentage of women diagnosed with this particular anemia. Pica can also afflict nonpregnant women and children. Pregnant women with pica crave and subsequently ingest unusual nonfood items, such as clay or dirt, or other items in large quantities, such as ice. There is no scientific understanding of the link between the behavior and the disease. Furthermore, if iron is added to the woman's diet and supplemented to the point of correcting the anemia, the pica symptoms, such as eating dirt or other strange substances, persists. We had a patient who craved the smell of rubber tires. She would go to Wal-Mart and gravitate to the car tire section just to inhale the scent of the tires. The craving became so intense that she would actually go to tire stores just because of the urge to smell the tires. This craving did not abate even when her anemia was corrected. She never gave in to eating the rubber, at least that she would admit. Why this occurred, we have no idea. Pica remains a medical enigma.

So, the bottom line is, if you are craving foods that are healthy, such as fresh fruits or vegetables or leaner meats, we recommend that you "give in" to your craving, in moderation, of course. If you crave junk food or fast food, try to find a healthy substitute that will equally satisfy you. If you start craving odd things like chalk or paint or rubber tires, consult your healthcare provider. There may be some underlying issue, such as anemia, that needs correcting.

4. You crave the foods that your baby wants to eat.

I remember when I was a little guy, sitting around the picnic table during Fourth of July festivities just loving the watermelon. My mom used to say that I loved watermelon even before I was born. I can remember looking at her like she was crazy.

"I ate watermelon almost every day I was pregnant," she would say.

"So?" I replied, juices and seeds running down my chin.

"You had me eating watermelon when you were still inside of me," she said more than once.

I remember thinking that was the weirdest thing I had ever heard. Was I always in love with watermelon and could I have somehow communicated this to my mother when she was pregnant with me? How would I have even known what watermelon tasted like if I was still inside of her belly? She seemed convinced that her craving for watermelon occurred because I craved watermelon during her pregnancy.

Patients tell us this all the time. They say things like "My baby must really love chocolate." There is no way to substantiate that scientifically, because you are separate entities, your baby and you. You have separate brains with separate desires and separate needs. There is most certainly a connection between mother and fetus both emotionally, spiritually, and physically. We believe that a mother's intuition is a true phenomenon. But maternal cravings that originate with the fetus is a difficult concept to take seriously, mainly because the fetus doesn't actually eat in utero (inside the womb). The baby growing inside of you gets all of its nutrition from your bloodstream, which flows into the placenta and then into the baby's bloodstream. The nutrition does not go into the baby's gastrointestinal tract at all, much less into the baby's mouth, where it would come in contact with its taste buds, which is where the satisfaction would occur. Even though cravings are not well understood, it's not likely they are dictated by the taste preferences or nutritional needs of your baby.

5. If I crave lighter-colored foods, my baby will have lighter-colored skin.

Skin color is contingent on the quantity of pigment in the layers of the skin. This pigment has nothing to do with the color in food; it has to do with your baby's genes. It is a genetic component, meaning it is encoded in your baby's chromosomes, which are components found in genes. When your egg and your partner's sperm meet, fertilization occurs and your baby's genetic code is set. It cannot change during your pregnancy. Thus, genetics determines the color of your baby's skin, not the food you ingest during pregnancy.

What about the baby who looks orange or yellow? We've all seen the baby who looks orange, right? Turns out that all he eats are carrots and sweet potato baby food. These particular foods are filled with a biochemical pigment called carotene. If eaten in large quantities, carotene can definitely alter a baby's skin color temporarily, but not permanently. When the same types of foods are eaten by a pregnant woman, this same pigment most definitely enters the bloodstream of the mother and crosses over the placenta to the fetal bloodstream. However, the levels are found to be much lower in the fetus as compared to the mother. So it seems it would take an impossibly large amount of ingested carotene to make any kind of significant skin color change, though we can't say for certain, since not enough studies have been done to eliminate this possibility.

Newborns do tend to get jaundice, a condition that turns their skin yellow, because of an increase in bilirubin, a by-product formed when red blood cells are broken down. The liver usually removes bilirubin from the bloodstream. The liver in newborns, however, is not fully developed and therefore is not as effective at the job as it needs to be. The bilirubin builds up and jaundice results. There are maternal conditions or diseases that can cause an infant to be born with an increase in bilirubin in its bloodstream, but those are not related to the mother's diet.

Rest assured, there is no way to alter the baby's skin color in utero, no matter what you eat. So even if you eat an abundance of darker foods, you won't give birth to a baby who looks like he just spent a week at the beach.

6. I heard that if I eat more breakfast cereal I will have a boy.

Really, can you imagine? Actually, there is some truth to this statement. In a study done in England regarding pre-pregnancy diets and their relation to the fetal gender, scientists found more boys born to women who ate a higher-calorie diet. More specifically, a higher percentage of boys were born to women who ate breakfast cereal each morning prior to becoming pregnant. The reason for this finding continues to be debated. When food, especially carbohydrates like breakfast cereal, is digested it turns into sugar. Research shows that a male fetus requires more energy to grow than a female fetus. One theory contends that the body can sense when its energy is running low and in an effort to conserve energy it makes a female fetus. Hence, eating more breakfast cereal before pregnancy begins may, and we strongly emphasize the word *may*, influence the gender of your baby. Eating breakfast cereal while pregnant, however, will not have an effect, since your baby's gender has already been determined.

7. If I crave meat and fizzy drinks, that means I am having a boy, and if I crave dairy products, it means I'm having a girl.

If boys are grouped into the category "snakes and snails and puppy dog tails," and girls in the category "sugar and spice, and everything nice," it wouldn't be a far stretch to connect meat, associated with the building of muscles, and "fizzy," with its association to high energy, with a boy. Likewise, it would make sense to connect dairy, much of which is milk based and comes from the female species, with a girl. How grounded is this myth in reality?

If you have never craved meat before, but crave it now that you're pregnant, your body probably needs iron. As for the carbonated, fizzy drinks, we tend to think you probably had similar cravings when you weren't pregnant. Now, with a baby in your belly, it could be that you are simply thirsty or slightly dehydrated and the carbonated beverages sound delicious. If you are craving the soda because of the sugar, then it would be advisable to switch to diet soda and limit the amount you drink to one or two servings per day. (We will address the pros and cons of diet sodas later.) In rare cases you may be craving regular soda, not so much for the fizz but because you may have diabetes and sugar is not getting into your tissues. Usually these cravings will be accompanied by other symptoms like frequent urination and an unquenchable thirst.

What if you crave dairy products?

First of all, there is a myth that you need to consume dairy products when you are pregnant in order to get the proper amount of vitamin D. The milk industry in this country and their genius marketing ads have us all believing that we need milk for strong bones, and since the baby inside of you is forming bones, then you must need to drink more milk, right? We are the only species of mammals that drinks milk outside of infancy, and the milk we drink is not human milk, it is bovine. Since the milk you're craving is cow's milk, does that mean you are having a baby cow? Of course not. Does that mean you're having a baby girl? No, it doesn't. There just isn't a connection. What your body is doing, in all its innate wisdom, is directing you to something you need. Most likely you're craving milk because you need the vitamin D and calcium. Other than iron, your prenatal vitamin should compensate for any deficiencies. The myth that cravings for milk products means you're having a girl probably developed because milk is a food your baby needs and only a woman can provide this type of nutrient to the developing baby. Remember, when you hear myths relating to gender in pregnancy, think back to the old Mother Goose nursery rhyme that associates boys with the rough and tumble and girls with sweet, nurturing traits.

8. Morning sickness means I will have a miscarriage or harm the baby in some other way.

Without a doubt, this one is pure myth. No one has to worry that morning sickness will cause a miscarriage, that you might vomit so hard that you'll push the baby out or do harm to it. Studies have shown women with morning sickness tend to have lower rates of miscarriage and preterm labor. If you have morning sickness to the point where you're vomiting multiple times a day, the only way to harm your baby is if you become dehydrated or cannot consume adequate calories. Otherwise, the baby is in its own little environment called the "bag of water" and will be fine.

Two evolutionary biologists at Cornell University found that morning sickness may actually be a way for a pregnant woman to protect the baby inside of her. They claim that certain food aversions protect her from consuming substances that might damage the baby in some way.[1] After researching thousands of pregnancies, they determined the following information regarding morning sickness:

- Morning sickness tends to occur when the organs of your baby are developing between weeks six and eighteen. This is a very delicate time during the pregnancy and it seems that the body might be trying to limit your intake of potential carcinogens or other compounds that could affect fetal development.
- If you experience morning sickness, you are less likely to miscarry; women who also experience vomiting are less likely to miscarry than those women with simple nausea.
- Aversions to meats, fish, poultry, and eggs are most common. Before refrigeration became available, these foods were most likely to confer bacteria and possible infections. Many women also avoided strong-tasting vegetables and caffeine.
- In traditional societies that rely on plants low in phytochemicals as staples instead of meat products, especially corn, few or no women experienced morning sickness. Phytochemicals protect plants from disease and insects; they offer no nutritive value to humans.

For those of you who have morning sickness that isn't severe, there is little medical intervention that is available. Even though you might feel awful, your baby will be safe and unharmed. Simply trying to eat those foods that sound appealing is the best method of treating this temporary illness. Listen to your body and trust in it to guide you along. If you don't have morning sickness, this is not a sign that something is wrong. It is a time to relish feeling good and to enjoy your health.

9. I don't have to worry about my diet because I supplement with prenatal vitamins.

Although vitamins can supplement your diet, they should not replace the habit of eating well. In fact, if you are eating a diet rich in fruits and vegetables with sufficient protein, you probably have enough nutrients to sustain a healthy pregnancy. If you find yourself dipping into nonnutritive snacks, however, then consider investing in a prenatal vitamin.

What constitutes a good prenatal vitamin? You want a product that includes the most important vitamins and minerals, but not in extreme quantities. The table below is a guideline for certain vitamins and the upper limits of normal so that you can check the vitamin you were prescribed or what you purchased over the counter. Keep in mind that many of the companies manufacturing these prenatal vitamins use marketing campaigns targeted to your fears of not having a healthy, happy baby.

Table Vitamin and Mineral Guidelines[2]

Vitamins/Minerals	RDA (Recommended daily allowance)	Upper Limits (Levels higher not recommended)*
VITAMIN A	750–770 mcg	2,800–3,000 mcg
VITAMIN D	80–85 mg/d	1,800–2,000 mg/d
VITAMIN E	15 mg/d	800–1,000 mg/d
VITAMIN C	80–85 mg/d	1,800 –2,000 mg/d
THIAMINE (B1)	1.4 mg/d	Not determined
RIBOFLAVIN (B2)	1.4 mg/d	Not determined
NIACIN (B3)	18 mg/d	30–35 mg/d
PYRIDOXINE (B6)	1.9 mg/d	80–100 mg/d
FOLATE	600 mcg	800–1,000 mg
CALCIUM	1,000–1,300 mg/d	2,500 mg/d
IRON	27 mg/d	45 mg/d
ZINC	12 mg/d	45 mg/d

*It is never recommended to take more than twice the RDA and it is also recommended that you not take multiple supplements at the same time rather take one supplement that has multiple minerals and vitamins.

Sitting here writing this section reminds me of a forty-year-old photograph that I have of my mother and two aunts sitting in our living room breastfeeding their babies. The interesting thing is that they are all smoking cigarettes. I mention this to bring to light two facts. The first is that we have such a better grasp of health in this country than in years past. We are far more aware of what vitamins and minerals our bodies need, pregnant or not. Second, I grew up without major health issues or chronic disease, even with my mother smoking cigarettes (and probably ate white bread and other processed foods common to that era), though I did have multiple ear infections. But that's another story.

10. Vegetarians and vegans cannot get enough protein during pregnancy.

If you're a vegetarian or vegan (someone who doesn't eat meat, fish, or any animal products), your well-intentioned family and friends may be advising you that you'll need to eat meat, and in the case of vegans, eat dairy too, in order to get sufficient protein while pregnant. In either case, rest assured, you *can* get enough protein in your diet, and that fact has been scientifically supported. One study, for instance, showed that pregnant vegans consumed 65 grams of daily protein.[3] The recommended daily amount of protein in a meat-inclusive diet is 71 grams per day.[4] If you are a vegan or a vegetarian and you are eating good amounts of beans, soy, or tofu and you can supplement with soy milk, then chances are you are getting adequate amounts of protein for your pregnancy.

As far as basic minerals and vitamins needed during pregnancy, how can you make sure that you're getting adequate amounts? Vegans should shoot for 1,300 mg of calcium per day. Choose calcium-fortified natural orange juices and other juices, as well as foods supplemented with B12 and folate. You'll be able to synthesize your own vitamin D simply by allowing yourself some daily sun without sunscreen, in moderation, of course.[5] We also recommend that you take a supplement like flaxseed oil or eat one to two servings of walnuts or the actual flax seeds daily in order to consume the proper amount of healthy omega fatty acids, since you aren't getting them via foods like fish.

You may have a hard time finding an ob-gyn who has enough nutritional background for routine nutritional counseling, much less vegetarian or vegan nutritional recommendations. Consider asking for a referral to a nutritionist who is knowledgeable about vegetarian or vegan diets. If you are vegetarian or vegan, be extra conscious about the proteins, carbohydrates, and fats in your foods. Reed Mangels and the Vegetarian Resource Group have written a wonderful book, *The Dietician's Guide to Vegetarian Diets*, which includes a chapter on pregnancy and lactation.[6] It's a bit pricey, but worth a look.

11. You should drink whole milk when pregnant, especially if you are going to breastfeed.

Got milk? The National Dairy Council would have you believe that milk is necessary for strong bones and healthy teeth. Its brilliant marketing campaign features celebrities and their milk mustaches, extolling the virtues of milk. Of course, they never mention the many other ways to include calcium in your diet. So let us repeat our mantra: pregnant women do not *need* to drink milk. Now, let us explain it.

The common assumption is that you need calcium and lots of it because not only do you need to keep your bones strong, but you need to keep your baby's bones strong as well. Without a doubt, you need calcium, but before you run to pour a glass of milk, read on. The absorption of calcium into your cells requires the activity of another cell called the *osteoblast*. When you consume calcium, these osteoblasts will utilize it to help create more bone. At the same time this is happening, another cell called the *osteoclast* is busy breaking down and deporting calcium from the bone. It's kind of like a tug-of-war between these two types of cells.

The problem is that when new bone is created, 50 to 70 percent of the osteoblasts die in the process. Fortunately, they are protected by the hormone estrogen. Estrogen actually inhibits absorption of calcium into the cells and thus saves your osteoblasts so they can continue to generate new bone. The great thing during pregnancy is that your estrogen levels are elevated and thus prevent your bones from degenerating. Your body is an amazing machine. It also knows how much calcium to absorb in order to grow and protect bones. On average, about 200 mg is absorbed daily whether you consume 200 mg or 2,000 mg. Your body will not absorb extra calcium if it does not need it. Contrary to popular belief, the less milk consumed, the lower the rate of osteoporosis.[7] Countries that consume more milk have higher rates of osteoporosis.

Another argument made for drinking milk is that it is rich in vitamin D, which is essential to calcium absorption in the gut. The most important source of vitamin D is not milk—it is the sun. Good old sunlight is far more likely to satisfy your vitamin D requirement than food. If you live in an area where you can sit outside comfortably for ten to fifteen minutes without sunscreen, you can produce your own vitamin D. If you're more likely to develop frostbite or be drenched from rain, consider eating the following foods, all of which contain the recommended daily amount of vitamin D.

- 1 ½ cups of fortified breakfast cereal
- 1 ounce of salmon, uncooked
- 1 ½ ounces of tuna, canned in oil

If you like milk, go ahead and drink it, but don't feel as though you are required to do so because you are pregnant. Skim or low-fat is just as good as whole milk and has fewer calories.

12. Spicy foods will bring on labor.

This would be great if it were true. We could then advise you to go home and eat a delicious chicken burrito with extra-hot salsa and you would come back in labor. This myth may have originated from the fact that spicy foods can cause abdominal cramping. This abdominal pain occurs in the intestines and stomach. As you near the full term of your pregnancy, your uterus fills your abdominal cavity, which means the cramping may be mis-construed as the uterus contracting. More than a few women have stories about eating spicy food and within hours ending up in the labor and delivery ward, only to be sent home again because they were not yet in labor. Their stomach and intestines were contracting, not their uterus.

To the best of our knowledge, there is no evidence or research showing that cayenne pepper, red pepper, or jalapeno peppers cause uterine contractions. There is some evidence that spices like cayenne can help with pain and can stop bleeding. We remember hearing stories of midwives in Oklahoma using a cayenne pepper compound after delivery to help stop the bleeding from an episiotomy or vaginal laceration. These midwives packed the laceration with this cayenne compound, which sig-nificantly reduced bleeding and helped to ease the pain. We have pre-scribed a cayenne-based cream for vulvar pathologies and we can report that cayenne does take away pain, but the initial application is a doozie, about as hot as you would imagine cayenne would feel down there. There are many references to cayenne pepper (capsicum) on the Internet, but if you look at those references regarding labor, some claim that it is effective for starting labor and increasing the strength of contractions, while others claim that it helps stop menstrual cramps. Until more definitive research is done, using cayenne pepper as any type of treatment or therapy is not advised.

> When Angela, a twenty-seven-year-old patient in her first pregnancy, was one week from her due date, she inquired about a possible induction of labor, as she was very uncomfortable. Because it was a week before her due date, she was considered an elective induction, and we weren't able to schedule her for at least seven days. Disappointed, she left vowing that she would come into the hospital "in labor" before her induction date. I told her to keep her fingers crossed.
>
> Later that evening I received a phone call from a labor and delivery nurse who said that Angela had arrived with intractable nausea and vomiting and severe abdominal pain. There were no contractions on the baby monitor, and the baby's heart rate was perfect. I asked Angela if she had eaten anything unusual or if anyone else in her house was sick. I ordered labs and an ultrasound to rule out appendicitis or a gallbladder issue. All of her tests came back normal, so we hydrated her and gave her anti-nausea medication, and I called for a general surgery consult.
>
> About thirty minutes later I received a call from a very amused general surgeon who asked me if I recommended that all my patients drink Tabasco sauce to induce labor. He stated that the patient heard that if she mixed a small bottle of Tabasco sauce with water and drank the concoction, it would put her into labor within twenty-four hours. Obviously, this had to run its course. I went to see her and explained that we were going to keep her overnight. When I asked her why she told me that she hadn't eaten anything unusual (as I considered the bottle of Tabasco sauce unusual), she replied, "You asked me if I *ate* anything unusual." From that point on I always asked my patients if they have had anything unusual to eat *or* drink.

13. If I eat spicy foods my baby will have colic.

We had friends who had a baby with colic. We remember them describing the days and nights without sleep, and how at six weeks, it all ended and everyone was fine.

Colic is often defined as unexplained crying for three or more hours a day, three days a week for more than three weeks (do you see a trend here?). There is usually a specific time of day that is worse than others. A colicky baby may pass gas or stool at the end of the episode. Mayo Clinic lists the cause of infantile colic as unknown, even though a multitude of studies have tried to discover the root cause of this process. Researchers could have been looking for Bigfoot, because they would have had as much success. There are, however, some risk factors that can increase the incidence of infantile colic. It seems to occur with a higher rate in:

- mothers who smoke either during or after pregnancy
- formula-fed babies
- firstborn children

Factors that have been shown not to influence the incidence of baby colic include:

- Mom's diet during pregnancy or while breastfeeding

Spicy foods can cause colic in adults, but the digestion systems between you and your baby are completely separate. While your baby will get the breakdown products of the foods you eat, he or she does not consume the whole foods. So even if those chili peppers cause you gastric distress, they won't go through the baby's stomach and therefore won't challenge the baby's digestion in the same way.

14. I can't eat fish.

Is there anything more confusing than how much fish we are supposed to eat? It seems like the recommendations change almost daily, and there are camps on both sides of the issue. Fish is good to eat. Fish *is* healthy to eat, but there are certain fish that have high levels of mercury in their meat, and mercury is something to avoid, particularly since mercury consumption during pregnancy has been linked to developmental delays.

If you are a seafood lover and like the idea of giving your baby omega fatty acids through your diet, then consume the following fish two times a week. These fish have the lowest amounts of mercury.

- flounder
- haddock
- herring
- butterfish
- anchovies
- tilapia
- sardines
- freshwater trout

There are also fish that harbor very high levels of mercury. These fish are to be avoided during pregnancy at any level of consumption.

- grouper
- marlin
- orange roughy
- tilefish
- swordfish
- shark
- king mackerel

We may sound like a broken record when it comes to dietary items, but even with safe fish, take things in moderation. If you have any questions regarding fish consumption, you can look to the National Resources Defense Council at http://www.nrdc.org.

What are you supposed to do if you like sushi? The reason you want to avoid uncooked sushi is the same reason you wouldn't want to eat uncooked beef or pork. Uncooked food products carry bacteria, and these can cause harm to you and your baby if ingested. It would be better to eat fish low in mercury and cooked to the point that destroys bacteria.

15. I was at the deli and when I ordered a salami sandwich, the woman next to me said I shouldn't eat lunch meat.

This type of interaction is the reason we wrote this book. So many people out there become experts around pregnant women, and in cases such as this they may impose their altruistic views upon you. We call this type of advice a mental grenade, because the well-minded individual at the deli counter launched this information into your brain and it explodes with a million feelings and questions. We tell you to include a decent amount of protein in your diet, but then reduce your options. First we give concern about fish. Then lunch meats.

There are two reasons we can think of that deli meats might be dangerous to your pregnancy. If these meats have been unrefrigerated for a long period of time or left in the sun, they can become infected with a bacteria called *Listeria monocytogenes*. This bacteria will usually only affect individuals with a decreased immune response. However, the immune response in pregnant women is somewhat blunted as well. Therefore you carry a greater risk for this infection than the lady at the counter who isn't pregnant. In fact, pregnant women are twenty times more likely to get listeriosis than nonpregnant women; about one-third of all listeriosis cases occur during pregnancy. Listeria is found in soil and water and can be carried by animals that may not appear ill. The bacteria is killed by pasteurization or high heat, but certain meats like hot dogs can become infected before or after packaging. The Centers for Disease Control and Prevention has recommended guidelines for pregnant women with regard to listeriosis prevention. Their recommendations for pregnant women are as follows:

- Thoroughly cook all foods from animal sources.
- Wash raw vegetables before consuming, as they may become infected with listeria through contact with animal manure.
- Consume ready-to-eat foods as soon as possible.
- Wash all utensils used for cutting meats, cheeses, and vegetables after use.
- Do not eat hot dogs, luncheon meat, or deli meat unless they are reheated or steaming hot.
- Avoid refrigerated smoked seafood and instead opt for canned or shelf-stable smoked seafood.[8]

There is no screening test for listeria, so if you are having symptoms of fever or stiff neck, we encourage you to call your physician or provider so the appropriate tests can be ordered.

Another buzzword related to luncheon meat is nitrates. Nitrates are chemical preservatives added to items like hot dogs and luncheon meats to protect you from listeria and botulism. The bad news is that nitrates can turn into cancer-forming nitrosamines in our stomachs. This can be combated by consuming an antioxidant such as vitamin C with your hot dog. A better meal decision would be to avoid these carcinogens altogether by not eating foods that contain nitrates. This may be easier said than done, especially if you crave hot dogs.

16. My grandmother told me not to eat cheese because it will infect my baby.

Certain cheeses can be considered risky, just like hot dogs and luncheon meat, especially certain soft chesses. First, make sure the cheese you eat is made with pasteurized milk, because the pasteurization process kills listeria. If you can't tell whether or not a particular cheese is made with pasteurized milk, then you are better off avoiding it. Unpasteurized cheeses include brie, feta, Camembert, blue-veined cheese, and Mexican-style cheeses like queso blanco, queso fresco, and queso-Panela. Obviously hundreds of cheeses are safe to consume and in moderation will provide you and your baby with a solid, stinky source of protein.

17. A friend told me that I shouldn't drink diet sodas because of the risk of exposing my baby to artificial sweeteners.

There are so many things you shouldn't do while pregnant. How much of a purist do you want to be? If you don't want to expose your baby to possible toxins, then artificial sweeteners like aspartame and sucralose should be avoided and the drinks of choice would be more-natural beverages (not such a bad idea). If you suffer from a disorder called phenylketonuria (PKU), then you already know you are not supposed to consume aspartame because you lack the ability to digest the amino acid phenylalanine, always found in aspartame.

If you aren't a pregnancy purist and you would like to have a diet soda because you like the taste or want to cut calories, is aspartame safe to consume during pregnancy? To date, no study proves that aspartame has a negative influence on unborn children. We realize that books and Web sites discuss the evils of aspartame, but again, no definitive scientific evidence supports complete avoidance of artificial sweeteners. Almost any compound or chemical has a toxic level at which consumption is harmless. Look at cyanide. It's one heck of a nasty compound that is used to poison people and will kill when ingested at a certain level. Well, almonds contain cyanide. Before you abandon this healthy snack, know that you would have to consume hundreds of pounds of them in order to reach a toxic dose of cyanide.

Not to sound like a broken record, the key is moderation, moderation, moderation. Do you remember the 1976 made-for-television movie *The Boy in the Plastic Bubble* starring John Travolta? We tell our patients that when they become pregnant they don't have to live inside of a plastic bubble, sequestered away from life's activities. You don't have to hide from the world around you because you are pregnant and you don't have to let those around you build a bubble around you. You're pregnant, you're not broken.

Many of you will feel ridden with guilt because you ate something wrong or someone told you not to drink that diet soda and you drank it anyway. As we've seen, diet myths continue to prevail. Similarly, there are times when guilt can get the better of you and make you think that you've done something that could harm your baby or cause a miscarriage. Myths abound that support and encourage your fears. As with diet, the topic of miscarriage abounds with myths. To ease your worries and fears, and thus lighten your load, we'll move on and do some miscarriage myth busting.

Notes

1. S. M. Flaxman and P. W. Sherman, "Morning Sickness: A Mechanism for Protecting Mother and Fetus," *Quarterly Review of Biology* 75, no. 2 (200): 131.

2. http://pregnancy.about.com/gi/dynamic/offsite.htm?zi=1/XJ&sdn =pregnancy&cdn=parenting&tm=24&f=00&su=p284.9.336.ip_p504.1.336.ip_&tt =2&bt=0&bts=0&zu=http%3A//www.iom.edu/File.aspx%3FID%3D21372 (accessed January 6, 2009).

3. E. Carlson et al., "A Comparative Evaluation of Vegan, Vegetarian, and Omnivore Diets," *Journal of Plant Foods* 6 (1985): 89.

4. http://www.iom.edu/Object.File/Master/4/154/MACRO8pgFINAL.pdf (accessed January 30, 2009).

5. B. L. Specker, "Do North American Women Need Supplemental Vitamin D during Pregnancy or Lactation?" *American Journal of Clinical Nutrition* 59 (1994): Supplement.

6. R. Mangels et al., *The Dietician's Guide to Vegetarian Diets: Issues and Applications,* 2nd ed. (London: Jones and Bartlett Publishers, 2004), p. 301.

7. A.V. Schwartz et al., "International Variation in the Incidence of Hip Fractures: Cross-National Project on Osteoporosis for the World Health Organization Program for Research on Aging," *Osteoporosis International* 9, no. 3 (1999): 242.

8. http://www.cdc.gov/nczved/dfbmd/disease_listing/listeriosis_gi.html (accessed December 30, 2008).

Chapter Five

Miscarriage Misconceptions
The Loss of Guilt

In medical circles a miscarriage is any pregnancy that terminates prior to the twentieth week of gestation. You may hear medical people use the term *abortion*, which, in this context, is the same as *miscarriage*. Medical personnel call a miscarriage a *spontaneous abortion*, which is a completely different process than the *elective abortion* that is the cause of so much controversy. This chapter will be dedicated to the myths surrounding spontaneous miscarriage.

It has been estimated that 78 percent of conceptions fail to result in a live birth, with many of these being aborted at the time of a missed menses.[1] This same source reports that 62 percent of pregnancies spontaneously miscarry before the twelfth week. Most people are amazed at the high numbers of miscarriages each year. The reason more people are not aware of the high numbers of miscarriage is because most miscarriages happen when the woman is not even aware she was pregnant; she thinks that she was just late on her menses and then had a heavy period.

There are multiple factors that can lead to a miscarriage, and the interval between pregnancies does not seem to be one of them, although many patients feel this may be a cause. There are factors such as maternal and paternal age, smoking, fever early in pregnancy, heavy occupational lifting, and chlamydial infections. These have all been implicated. The frequency of chromosomal abnormalities in aborted tissues ranges from 30 to 60 percent.[2] In this sense the miscarriage is an evolutionary system put in place so as not to propagate babies with multiple medical maladies or issues not compatible with life.

When a couple experiences miscarriage, they have questions about why it happened and how to prevent it in the future. The presence of abnormal chromosomes seems to be the most common reason for miscarriage. The means to effectively reduce the rate of miscarriage in the general population is unknown at this point. Studies on women who have experienced three or more miscarriages have not revealed any discernable means of prevention in the group. The take-home message we attempt to convey to these patients is that, in most cases, there is nothing that could have been done to prevent the miscarriage and there is nothing they did to cause it. Here are some myths and superstitions surrounding miscarriage. It is our hope that couples reading this book who have gone through a miscarriage will understand that sometimes such things are left to something bigger than all of us.

1. I can stop a miscarriage from happening.

As discussed earlier, the main cause for a miscarriage is that of chromosomal anomalies of the fetus. So what are the myths regarding the cause of miscarriage, and can any of them be avoided or prevented?

- **Miscarriage can be caused by stress.** There are people on both sides of the fence on this issue. A small study done in 2006 showed an increased rate of miscarriage in women with elevated levels of the stress hormone cortisol. Researchers and academicians are excited by this finding because it is measurable and can be followed. The problem with the study is that stress can be caused by a multitude of issues, so it isn't known at what levels the miscarriages were found. Of note, there were pregnant women who lost spouses during the September 11, 2001, attacks on the World Trade Center; to the best of our knowledge, these women went on to deliver healthy babies, and no one would argue the high-stress levels surrounding this event. There are currently studies being done on the aftermath of 9/11 on pregnant women and children that were exposed to the chaos. If we assume that there is a link between stress and miscarriage, then women are obviously upset by the fact that many providers will simply tell them to relax. This is a difficult topic to discuss with patients because of the multitudes of religious and spiritual backgrounds. While some women may practice yoga and mindfulness, some may choose contemplative thought or some other religious teaching. It would be beneficial to the treatment of stress during pregnancy if physicians were trained to ask patients about their spiritual backgrounds. It is only when we know patients' backgrounds that we can hopefully make a difference in their lives. It is appropriate for physicians to become more familiar with the spiritual aspects of their patients and realize that medicine is indeed multicultural. Nowhere has the connection between spirituality and medicine been better documented than in Anne Fadiman's book *The Spirit Catches You and You Fall Down*. In this book one reads about the medical community trying desperately to help a young Hmong child with a perceived seizure disorder and a family who feels the child is suffering from a spiritual crisis or that she is being called from this earth to greater things. The physicians and social workers have the child removed from her parents, and the young child eventually dies.[3] The disconnect between the physician and the patient in the case of miscarriage and stress is shown not only in the fact that physicians do not have an understanding of patients and their spiritual history, but the physicians themselves are stressed beyond reason.

- **If I stop lifting my other children, this will reduce my risks.** Lifting in later pregnancy should be limited to ten to twenty pounds. A good rule of thumb is to monitor your breathing, and if you have to hold your breath in order to pick something up, then it is probably too heavy and you should ask for help. Personally, we would not recommend for any pregnant women to lift items that cause severe strain on the body, but this might be unavoidable for women who work in physically demanding jobs. In those cases, we would say, lift with your legs. If you can't pick it up with your knees bent then ask for help; chivalry has not completely died.

- **Now that I'm pregnant, if I want to prevent a miscarriage I need to stop working out.** Please don't use pregnancy as an excuse not to exercise. Getting your heart rate up a bit is great for you and your baby. It would be helpful to take your pulse every so often or buy a heart rate monitor and not allow your pulse to stay over 140 beats per minute for extended periods of time. Remember, this is not a weight loss program, it's a pregnancy.

- **I can cause a miscarriage if I continue to eat fast food.** Shawn would use any excuse to eat at In-N-Out Burger, but the simple fact is that the typical American diet is laden with partially hydrogenated oils, fat, and carbohydrates. While eating poorly may not be the best thing for your baby, it is hardly a crime and will not cause a miscarriage. One patient of ours craved Burger King so frequently she would hide the empty bags at the bottom of the trash can. If you find yourself digging to the bottom of your trash can in order to hide the wrapper of some chocolate-laden treat or hamburger, stop and ask yourself why. Be proud of your girth and know that the cravings will go away.

- **I had a few drinks before I even knew I was pregnant; will this cause a miscarriage?** You have been trying to get pregnant for eight months. After a night out with your girlfriends (and yes, you did a pregnancy test earlier in the day, just to make sure, and it was negative), you wake up the next morning and run to the toilet bowl, wishing you hadn't hung out with Captain Morgan and Lady Tequila the night before. The thought then suddenly crosses your mind that you might be pregnant and you quickly muster up enough urine from your dehydrated body to pee on the stick. Lo and behold, the line turns blue. Has this ever actually happened? Sure. Did these women go on to deliver happy, healthy babies? I am sure many did. The point is that a miscarriage occurs because there is something terminally wrong with the genetic makeup or there is an acute, devastating assault like chemotherapy that affects the fetus. Alcohol can indeed cause fetal alcohol syndrome if a pregnant woman consumes one to two drinks a day for an extended period of time during the pregnancy. Patients at high risk are those who have blood alcohol levels over 100 mg/dl delivered to the fetus at least weekly during the pregnancy.[4]

2. I am bleeding in my first trimester and this means I am going to have a miscarriage.

Sheila was a twenty-five-year-old bank attendant who had recently found out she was pregnant. Like most women, she didn't want to tell people she was pregnant until she was about eleven or twelve weeks along, for fear of everyone getting excited and then possibly having to tell them she miscarried. She had been having slight amounts of spotting throughout the early portion of the first trimester; in medical terms, this is called a *threatened abortion.* We had told her that about 40 percent of all pregnancies will have some spotting or bleeding in the first trimester and that more than half of these will go on to be normal. Obviously, bleeding during pregnancy is scary and is one of the main reasons we receive calls in the middle of the night. We ordered an ultrasound for Sheila and saw a little baby nugget about nine weeks along with a beautiful heart rate. The heart rate is significant for multiple reasons, but when it's seen during an ultrasound it can be very reassuring. Women whose ultrasounds show a visible or audible fetal heart rate in the first trimester have a miscarriage rate of less than 3 percent. Sheila felt she could tell her friends and family at this point because she had a 97 percent chance that things would be just fine. While bleeding can indeed be the harbinger of bad news, it is not necessarily a cause for alarm.

3. Cramping in early pregnancy is a sign of miscarriage.

What makes you cramp? Well, let's see, what is in your pelvis? Early in pregnancy there are a multitude of things that can cause cramping. The structures of the pelvis that can cause this sensation are uterus, ovaries, bladder, bowel, muscle, and tendons. In the first ten weeks of pregnancy the uterus is expanding and swelling larger than it has ever been (if this is your first pregnancy). This stretching and growth can cause some minor irritability and cramping in the uterus. In addition, one of the ovaries will have the *corpus luteum cyst* of pregnancy, and this can cause a cramping sensation on one side of the lower abdomen. Constipation from increased progesterone levels can cause a fullness and cramping sensation in the lower pelvis, and bladder infections can also create feelings of cramping in the pelvis. None of these problems would necessarily be attributed to miscarriage, but the sensation of cramping can definitely be related to miscarriage. We usually recommend that if you are experiencing severe cramps and/or heavy bleeding (heavier than during a normal menses), you should call your physician immediately or proceed to the emergency room. Overall, cramping during the first trimester of pregnancy is a common occurrence and can happen for many reasons, most of which are not a threat to the pregnancy.

4. I am pregnant, but I don't feel pregnant; this must be a bad sign.

Does every woman have sore breasts, nausea, bloated belly, and constipation in early pregnancy? Thankfully, no—what a horrible world that would be. The problem with "feeling pregnant" is that everyone feels the effects of pregnancy differently. The following list from *Obstetrics: Normal and Problem Pregnancies*[5] describes some of the normal side effects and symptoms of pregnancy that one might expect:

- **Appetite.** You may experience an increased appetite starting early in the first trimester and possibly extending into the latter portion of the pregnancy—assuming you aren't throwing up every five minutes. You may even want to eat crazy things like dirt, coal, or toothpaste. If you don't have a craving to eat newspaper, not to worry, a simple mild increase in appetite is normal.
- **Constipation.** You may feel constipated because of the colon increasing its absorption of water, the uterus obstructing the stool moving out of the rectum, and the decreased movement of the colon. Hopefully you are drinking at least eight glasses of water a day. We ask our patients to remember the "golden" rule: If your urine is golden, then you're not drinking enough water. We realize that after you take your prenatal vitamin your urine is an ectoplasmic yellow, but later in the day, if you are properly hydrated, the urine should be fairly clear.
- **Morning sickness.** This typically occurs on an empty stomach, which for most women is in the morning and thus the reason for the

name. Morning sickness occurs in 70 percent of pregnancies, so that means there are 30 percent of you out there wondering why you aren't vomiting. Typically the sickness lasts from the first four to fourteen weeks. The reason many women worry if they are not sick is because of the myth that a pregnancy with good levels of hormones will make you sick. There does not seem to be a connection between the maternal levels of pregnancy hormone human chorionic gonadotropin and the degree of nausea and vomiting. This means you can have your cake and eat it too... well, at least 30 percent of you can.

- **I can't catch my breath.** The sensation of shortness of breath will occur in 60 to 70 percent of normal pregnancies in the late first trimester; that means 30 to 40 percent will not have this sensation. This does not account for those women with asthma. If you have asthma, remember to take your medications as needed. Breathing is a very important part of pregnancy. We have patients ask us if they need to use their inhalers, and I remind them that breathing is essential.

- **I can't hold it any longer.** Most women will experience the need to urinate more frequently once they are pregnant. As the blood volume increases during pregnancy the kidneys are responsible for filtering more waste, making you pee more frequently. If you are already used to drinking large amounts of water during the day, you may not notice an increased need to visit the bathroom.

- **Bionic breasts.** We had a patient who was only ninety-five pounds in the early portion of her pregnancy, and her breasts went from an A cup to a C cup in a matter of months. This was an obviously dramatic change in her appearance and one of the reasons her friend (also pregnant) asked if there was something wrong with her own pregnancy, because her breasts did not attain the same quick growth. We reassured the friend that breast growth is a response to increased blood flow and that breasts can change from 0 to 800 ml with the average being about 200 ml (little more than a half can of soda). We also told her that her breasts would continue to enlarge with breastfeeding, but that she needed to remember that breast size decreases after breastfeeding; what goes up must come down.

- **I need new contacts.** Depending on the shape of your eyes, you may need to have them examined, because changes in the corneas due to fluid retention can be cause for your prescription to change. The change in the eyes is only about 3 percent, so for most women this will not be a noticeable change. For those who have been putting off changing that prescription for years, however, they may need to have things looked at … literally.

5. If I am having a miscarriage, that means I did something wrong.

We have discussed that many pregnancies will miscarry and that the number one reason is a genetic mistake when sperm and egg unite. One of the hardest things to see is a woman who feels as though she has done something to cause the pregnancy to miscarry. Assuming that you are not using illicit drugs or undergoing chemotherapy in the first trimester, there are a multitude of reasons to miscarry that are simply not in your control.

> KA came to the office in a panic because she was eight weeks pregnant with her second child and the evening before she had gone to the emergency room for an asthma attack. They had done an x-ray of her chest (remember, breathing is important), and she was concerned that the x-ray may have been the reason for her to have a miscarriage. Her belly was shielded with a lead apron, so there was no need for concern, but it is easy to understand how she would have been worried under the circumstances.

Women undergo surgery, trauma, x-rays, and illnesses when they are pregnant, and most of these situations will not affect the pregnancy unless they are of such significance they cause damage to the mother.

If you have had the sad experience of miscarriage, please do not blame yourself. Try to understand that in most cases, this is nature's way of protecting us, although it may not seem like it at the time. Most women who experience a miscarriage go on to become pregnant again and have successful pregnancies. Before you go down the road of condemning yourself for something you might have done, make an appointment with your physician and ask as many questions as you need to in order to feel better. This is not a time for blame. It is a time to heal.

6. I have had a miscarriage and I heard it is bad to get pregnant again right away.

Normally, we recommend that you wait a few months and have two or three normal menses before you attempt pregnancy again. This recommendation is not based on cold hard science. First of all, we want to make sure that the hormones from the miscarriage have gone back down to normal and that all the tissue has been removed from the uterus. This can be done with simple blood tests. Once this chemical is gone from the bloodstream, your body no longer has the signal that it is pregnant and your brain can then begin communicating with the ovaries to start up the process for ovulation and a menstrual cycle. Our concern for women who try for pregnancy immediately after a miscarriage or right after coming off of birth control is that the body may not have enough time to get ramped up again for a pregnancy. Some older studies have shown that there is no disadvantage to becoming pregnant immediately after a miscarriage, but we feel that this could be an emotionally hard time for your family and the stress endured could be detrimental. Allowing yourself a few months to get back into a normal rhythm for you, your spouse, and family may help decrease stress levels. We know there will be a bit of anxiety with the next pregnancy and the concern for another miscarriage is high, but rest assured, in most cases the rates for miscarriage are not elevated if you have had one miscarriage. This leads to the next myth.

7. My chances of miscarriage are higher because I have already had one miscarriage.

If you have had one miscarriage, then your chances of miscarriage during the second pregnancy are not increased. If you have had more than one miscarriage, however, the rate does increase. The short list below shows how the rates are figured based on the number of miscarriages and the age of the mother:

- Two prior miscarriages—20 percent rate in next pregnancy
- Three prior miscarriages—40 percent rate in next pregnancy

- Four prior miscarriages—54 percent rate in next pregnancy
- Maternal age thirty to thirty-nine—25 percent rate of miscarriage
- Maternal age forty to forty-four—50 percent rate of miscarriage
- Maternal age forty-five and over—approximately 95 percent rate of miscarriage[6]

There are other risk factors for miscarriage that have been discussed already. Drinking more than five alcoholic beverages weekly while pregnant increases the risk of miscarriage by fourfold, while obesity may increase miscarriage rates by half.

8. If I miscarry, there will be a large workup to find out why.

In most cases, if you have one or two miscarriages we do not perform an extensive workup to discover the reason. This is because in the majority of cases there is no immediate reason; it simply happened by chance. When a woman has three or more miscarriages, she is diagnosed with chronic habitual abortion, and the work is then started. It is our responsibility to provide you with the recurrence risks for miscarriage and help you to realize that not every couple requires an extensive workup. If you are an infertile couple in your forties, we would consider a workup sooner because of the advanced risks and decreased time frames. If you have had three losses or more, we would definitely recommend that testing be done. If you have undergone only one pregnancy that resulted not in a miscarriage but a stillborn infant, we would recommend genetic testing of the infant and both parents to help determine a cause. Genetic anomalies are the most common reason for miscarriage, and it is true for those with recurrent miscarriage issues. Other factors that can lead to recurrent miscarriage are thyroid abnormalities, diabetes mellitus, intrauterine scar tissue, fibroids of the uterus, infection, incompetent cervix (inability of the cervix to hold the pregnancy), blood disorders, and serious drug or alcohol abuse.

Notes

1. D. A. Grimes, "Management of Abortion," in *TeLinde's Operative Gynecology* (New York: Lippincott Raven, 1997), p. 477.

2. Ibid., p. 478.

3. A. Fadiman, *The Spirit Catches You and You Fall Down* (New York: Farrar, Straus, and Giroux, 1998).

4. http://www.surgeongeneral.gov/pressreleases/sg02222005.html (accessed January 5, 2009).

5. S. G. Gabbe, J. L. Simpson, and J. R. Niebyl, eds., *Obstetrics: Normal and Problem Pregnancies*, 5th ed. (New York: Churchill Livingstone, 2007).

6. L. J. Heffner, "Advanced Maternal Age: How Old Is Too Old?" *New England Journal of Medicine* 351 (2004): 1927.

Chapter Six

Mood and Behavior Myths
Women Behaving Badly

I
f you tuned in to the *Today Show* on June 23, 2005, you would have witnessed the interchange between host Matt Lauer and actor Tom
Cruise, during which Cruise criticized actress Brooke Shields for using
antidepressants to deal with her postpartum depression. That day, our
clinic received more than a few phone calls from pregnant and postpartum
patients taking medications for various mental health issues. The callers
wanted to know if it was true that they shouldn't be on these medicines.
They wanted to know what was fact and what was fiction. As with every
other aspect of pregnancy, myths and superstitions surround the moods
and behaviors common in pregnancy.

Pregnancy is not only a time of physical transition but also of emotional and mental transition. Your mental health is an essential component
of your experience. Women struggling with mood and other mental health
issues during and after pregnancy need to know the facts about conditions
such as mood swings, anxiety, depression, and postpartum blues. Celebrities and other public figures may mean well when they dispense advice, but
often it's not correct. So let's set the record straight about some of these
issues.

Mood swings during pregnancy can be mild and unobtrusive or, as one

93

patient described, "like a pendulum swinging between heaven and hell." Any discussion of moods should not only address feelings like sadness or joy but also should examine behavior. How do you behave when you are caught in a particular mood? Some women with anxiety or depression comfort themselves by eating excessively, while others can't bring themselves to eat anything. Some will pick up the cell phone and talk for hours. Others will rely on medication to ease their symptoms. Moods instigate behaviors. So what are some common moods and resulting behaviors, and what are the myths and superstitions of how they affect you, your pregnancy, and your baby?

1. **I'm so anxious and worried about the baby,
    about delivering . . . the list seems long.
    All I do is eat. But then again I'm pregnant,
    so it's okay, because most of the extra pounds
    will be from the baby.**

What do we do at every office visit? We make you step on the scale. We can't say how many times a day we hear patients say, "I hate this part," but it does help us track how much weight gain can be attributed to the baby and how much to conditions such as edema (fluid retention) or overeating.

If you're anxious and eat to assuage your anxiety, you might end up consuming too many calories and gaining unneeded pounds. Finding methods to deal with stress issues involving food is in your and your baby's best interest. You might consider, for example, joining a support group of other pregnant women. Or you might sign up for a yoga class or learn how to meditate. If your anxiety feels insurmountable and food becomes a regular antidote, talk to your healthcare provider. He or she may suggest that you get some counseling to help you manage your worries.

Currently we recommend that women of average weight gain between twenty-five and thirty-five pounds during a normal pregnancy. For women who are underweight, a weight gain of up to forty pounds is acceptable; overweight women should try to limit weight gain to fifteen pounds; morbidly obese patients really do not need to gain weight.

One of our patients started her pregnancy at 402 pounds. At the midpoint in her pregnancy (twenty weeks), she had gained eight pounds and she was seriously concerned that she was not gaining enough weight. I had a long talk with her about the needs of the baby and the excess weight that she was carrying daily. I told her I was not concerned that she was not gaining enough weight and, in fact, might even benefit from losing a small amount of weight. She was upset with my assessment and felt that I was wrong because she thought that all pregnant women were supposed to gain weight. This is one of the current myths of pregnancy. The truth is, a woman's weight gain during pregnancy depends on her weight at the time of conception.

What part of your weight gain relates directly to the baby? The answer depends on how much weight you actually gain. Keep in mind that your body is preparing to breastfeed, and since most of what makes up breast milk is fat, your body will want to pack on some extra fat prior to the delivery. The good news is that if you breastfeed, you will also burn extra calories.

Here is a breakdown of the weight that you will lose at delivery:

- 2–3 pounds of amniotic fluid
- 3–4 pounds for increased blood volume
- 1–2 pounds for breast enlargement
- 2 pounds due to the increased size of the uterus
- 6–8 pounds for the infant
- 1–2 pounds for the placenta

If you have a seven-pound baby, then approximately twenty pounds of weight gain is lost within weeks of the delivery. That leaves about six to eight pounds of maternal fat stores. These fat stores will be used quickly by your hungry baby during breastfeeding.

What you don't want is to gain an enormous amount of weight (fifty to sixty pounds) because then you are looking at about thirty pounds not related to the baby and possibly sticking around after you finish breastfeeding. As we mentioned above, in some cases, you can't control the amount of weight gain, especially if you retain excessive amounts of fluid in your feet and legs, but in most cases weight gain is controllable by eating a healthy diet and including mild to moderate exercise.

2. My husband is gaining weight because of my pregnancy.

In many cases, your husband will gain weight during your pregnancy because he is eating with you. Perhaps you're eating more comfort foods that are higher in calories than your usual diet. If he's consuming these foods, he, too, is ingesting more calories and could be packing on extra pounds. Or maybe you're both just eating more healthy food. While you have a reason to gain twenty-five to thirty-five extra pounds, he doesn't. Most men are not consciously aware that they are eating more and gaining weight. It's as if they are subconsciously trying to support you by gaining weight themselves. The problem is that he doesn't really have an excuse to have a pregnant-looking belly, and you do.

Also remember that your husband will play a peripheral role during your pregnancy. After all, it is your pregnancy. A study done in England in 2007 looked at 281 males with pregnant wives and compared them to married men whose wives weren't pregnant. These researchers found that a majority of men with pregnant spouses had pregnancy-associated symptoms such as morning sickness and mood swings. The most common symptom for the man with a pregnant wife was stomach cramps. One husband even had pains rivaling those of his laboring wife. (Wonder if he received an epidural?) Eleven of the men in the study reported going to the physician for their ailments, and in all these cases there were no reported diagnoses.

In general, the men experienced their pains at the same time their wives experienced similar symptoms. Your husband, for instance, may be inclined to experience morning sickness during your first trimester—the point when you are likely to experience morning sickness. This type of sympathetic pregnancy condition is called Couvade syndrome and has been reported to affect up to 65 percent of men with pregnant spouses.

When a man or woman appears to be pregnant with a swollen abdomen but is not pregnant, the disorder is called pseudocyesis. Women with pseudocyesis actually may test positive for pregnancy even though they're not pregnant; they may even have a softening of the cervix and labor pains. The symptoms can last for a few months to nine months and even longer. Couvade syndrome and pseudocyesis have been reported in men, as well as sisters and female friends of pregnant women. In our clinic, we've seen a number of cases of Couvade syndrome.

Grace was a twenty-seven-year-old mother of two and was in for her third pregnancy. Her husband, also young, and very supportive of his wife, accompanied her on every visit. A painter, he was finding it hard to stay working in the weakened economy and was starting to feel the financial pinch. He always came to the office in his painter's pants and shirt looking like a splatter of color. He rarely had any questions, so I was intrigued one day when he asked me if I could stay and answer a personal question for him. I have to admit that as a gynecologist, I'm not good with male issues, but I thought it might possibly be a "dad" question. He pulled up his shirt and showed me his belly. He said that hardly any of his work clothes were fitting, and he was also having issues climbing up onto a ladder, because he was having lower back pain. I looked back at his wife and then at him again and noticed that they looked the same. Each had a little pooch consistent with a twenty-week pregnancy. I advised him to get evaluated by his primary care doctor, who might order an x-ray of his belly to make sure there wasn't anything going on in there. His wife said, "He's trying to steal my thunder. He wants to be pregnant so he can get some time off of work." He sat down and rubbed his belly. "That would be nice," he admitted. "It's okay," she said, "if you go ahead and push this baby out from your butt with no anesthesia, agree to feed it at night, and change most of the diapers. Then it's okay for you to be pregnant." He slowly stood up and walked out the door. His wife looked at me and said, "I thought so."

Sometimes during a pregnancy, the husband is left on the outside looking in. If you have children already, he may take a backseat to them. Pretty soon he may begin to feel that his needs are not being met. It is a difficult time for you to have to take care of your kids, pregnancy, and the biggest baby of them all, your husband. We can almost guarantee that he will respond to a little TLC. Give it a try. Maybe you do something special for him and then the two of you make a pact to do something for each other once a week. Or make time to spend with him and share your worries and concerns. Many of your worries and concerns are likely the same as his.

3. My friend just told me that increased cell phone use can hurt my baby. I'm concerned because I frequently use my cell phone, especially since we no longer have a home phone.

Boy, did this topic ever hit the proverbial fan in 2008 when a group of researchers concluded that cell phone usage during pregnancy may increase behavioral problems in babies.[1] As national media reported, the study surveyed 13,000 women who used cell phones two to three times per day. The resulting data indicated that the more a woman talks on her cell phone while pregnant, the more likely it is that her child will be hyperactive or have other emotional and behavioral issues. The study's accuracy, however, has come under scrutiny for a number of reasons.

One of the problems is that researchers also took into consideration the child's use of cell phones through age seven. Thus, it's difficult to attribute with certainty a child's hyperactivity to in utero exposure to cell phones. Could that child's use of a cell phone also contribute to or aggravate behavioral and emotional issues? Some skeptics feel that women who talk excessively on the phone may be more inclined to ignore the needs of their children, a factor that explains why the incidence of hyperactivity among these children was higher. Another flaw with this study is that it was conducted via a survey—not always the most reliable method, because some people will take the time to do the survey and some will not. The interviewers found that women with hyperactive children were more likely to fill out the study than those who did not have hyperactive children. The resulting data may have been unfairly weighted. Finally, a number of other published studies show that cell phones do not pose an increased risk during pregnancy.

So if you were watching CNN on May 21, 2008, you heard the anchorperson tell you to limit usage of your cell phone if you are pregnant. Chances are you might have called your obstetrician, who claimed he had never heard of that, and with good reason: there currently is no recommendation claiming that women should limit their usage of cell phones. The CDC has found no link between cell phone use and problems with pregnancies, but the question is whether or not the child will have developmental issues after birth. More studies need to be undertaken.

For now, we feel it a good precaution to decrease your belly's exposure to cell phones. This means setting the phone away from you and using the speaker option if possible or using an ear apparatus like a wireless Bluetooth headset.

4. If I'm weepy and fatigued after delivering, I have postpartum depression.

Weepiness and fatigue following delivery is not all that unusual, but it does not necessarily indicate that you have postpartum depression. You could have a case of postpartum blues, which has different characteristics than postpartum depression.

Postpartum depression usually begins within four weeks of delivery and involves symptoms of major depression. Excessive feelings of hopelessness, loss of pleasure in daily activities, uncontrollable crying, severe anxiety, fatigue, sleep problems, and appetite change are common symptoms of depression. A woman suffering postpartum depression also may be overly preoccupied with her infant's safety or, on the other hand, may have complete disinterest in her baby or even have thoughts of harming her baby. Singer and actress Marie Osmond describes such an emotional state in her book *Behind the Smile: My Journey out of Postpartum Depression.* "I feel like I am playing hide and seek from my own life, except that I just want to hide and never be found. I want to escape my body. I don't recognize it anymore. I have lost my resemblance to my former self. I can't laugh, enjoy food, sleep, concentrate on work, or even carry on a conversation. I don't know how to go on feeling like this; the emptiness, the endless loneliness. Who am I? I can't go on."[2]

There have been questions as to whether or not postpartum depression is caused by lower estrogen levels. While one study showed that replacing estrogen in the postpartum period decreased the incidence of depression by 50 percent, later studies have failed to replicate these results. Many factors can contribute to postpartum depression, particularly a personal or family history of depression or bipolar disorder. If you suffer from depression prior to becoming pregnant, you will not necessarily experience postpartum depression. It's best to work with your caregiver to address this issue in advance.

Postpartum depression differs from the milder postpartum blues. Postpartum blues may affect between 50 to 70 percent of postpartum women. It's considered to be a temporary state of sadness, anxiety, fatigue, and confusion possibly caused by the sharp drop in estrogen. Postpartum blues will usually occur within a few days of the delivery and will subside within two to three weeks. Postpartum depression, on the other hand, has much more severe symptoms and may last seven months or longer. One of the most significant reasons for prolonged postpartum depression is a delay in being treated for the disease. As physicians, we want to be involved immediately. Sometimes this means beginning treatment for depression prior to delivery. One study published in the *British Medical Journal* reported that 25 percent of postpartum depression cases began during pregnancy.[3]

Never hesitate to share how you're feeling with your caregiver. We're here to help you heal and enjoy every aspect of motherhood as much as possible.

5. My mom told me to calm down because my angry outbursts and mood swings can hurt my baby.

Are you mad?

Have you yelled at someone today?

Are you concerned that this will hurt your baby?

Rest assured that your anger, happiness, and fatigue usually will affect only you. Although you and your baby are one, you also are separate. Your baby is a separate functional unit, and unless you are physically putting yourself in harm's way there is little that you can do to hurt your unborn child.

Understand, however, that your baby might be able to hear by the twenty-third week of gestation and will respond to angry outbursts with movement. Recent research indicates that infants will decrease movements after being exposed to soothing sounds such as the music of Beethoven and will increase movements when exposed to more stimulating sounds such as loud rock music. In later stages of pregnancy, the loud sounds of emotional conversations can be heard by the baby, and just like a baby jumps in her crib at the sound of loud noises, she will jump when startled in utero.

If you are prone to extreme emotional outbursts or live with someone who is and there is a chance of bodily harm to either you, your spouse, or the baby, then we would recommend you immediately call 911. If you find yourself becoming angry at the slightest provocation, consult your physician or healthcare provider. Asking for assistance is the best method of approach if you find yourself becoming increasingly angry or anxious. Yelling at your children should be reserved for their teenage years. Just kidding, of course.

6. Although my husband isn't gaining weight with me, my moods are affecting him.

There is no doubt that an extended period of minor depressive symptoms can affect those around you. If you notice that your husband is mirroring your moods, try a change of venue. Plan a trip or even a half-day outing with him, or try to get him out of the house with his buddies. "Man time" with his friends might be just what the doctor ordered. A round of golf or a night out with the boys might be enough to infuse him with the energy to elevate his mood. It's always our hope that you will stay open to talking about problems, fears, and other issues with your partner, family, and friends, as they may have helpful advice or just gentle reassurance that all is well.

7. I'm in the mood for sex, but since I'm pregnant, I need to abstain so that the baby doesn't get hurt.

I would venture to say that most men would quickly say this statement is all myth, coauthor of this book included. Speaking from a medical standpoint, these men are correct. The only reason to abstain from intercourse during pregnancy is if you develop any of the following conditions: placenta previa, in which the placenta develops in front of the cervix; preterm labor; bleeding; or an incompetent (weakened) cervix that requires a surgical procedure called cervical cerclage. During this procedure, the cervix is actually stitched closed to prevent miscarriage or premature delivery. During intercourse, if the penis bumps or rubs the cervix, it could dislodge the stitching, so it's best to avoid penetration. Otherwise, sex is safe during pregnancy.

Perhaps your sex drive will increase when you're pregnant, and then your husband can thank his lucky stars. It has been our experience that women are usually most sexually active during the second trimester. Many women lose their sex drive during the first trimester due to nausea or vomiting, tender breasts, or increased fatigue, none of which tend to encourage feelings of arousal. The second trimester is usually when you're feeling your best. Sex during the third trimester is definitely safe but can be awkward with a protruding tummy. We can reassure you that most sexual practices are completely safe.

So what *isn't* safe during pregnancy? One unsafe practice is your partner blowing into your vagina while performing oral sex. Because of the increased blood flow to the vagina and uterus, a certain amount of air can get into the bloodstream and could cause a potentially fatal air embolism. Our advice: If you are blessed with the opportunity to have sex with your partner, don't let him blow it.

A second unsafe practice is not knowing the sexual history of your partner. I hope your partner is close to you and has been open with you about his past partners. Unfortunately, many women who do contract chlamydia or gonorrhea infections in pregnancy have been sexually active only with their current partner. These men, if ever seen again, are found clutching an old VHS tape of the Farrah Fawcett revenge movie *The Burning Bed*. All kidding aside, sexually transmitted diseases are a real problem in our society. Diseases such as HIV and hepatitis not only affect the mother, they can be transmitted to the innocent fetus, so be cautious.

Sometimes a patient, or more likely the patient's partner, will wonder if her partner's penis can physically injure the unborn baby. Well, let's take a moment to discuss genitalia and that age-old question if size matters.

Some studies have shown that the average male penis is anywhere from five to seven inches in length when fully erect. The average vagina can accommodate at least nine inches of penis. Let us not forget that the vagina is also capable of accommodating an eight-pound baby. Occasionally during intercourse, the penis may hit the cervix, which is the lower part of the uterus that dilates during the first part of labor. If the cervix is closed and thick, then even if the fully erect penis pokes into it, there will be no trauma to the mother or baby. As much as your partner may feel macho by thinking he might poke the baby, most likely he's not even getting close to the cervix.

We've had couples ask if the baby is getting bumped on the head during sex. When the penis bumps the cervix, it is assumed that the penis is hitting the poor baby in the head. Over and over, the penis is hitting the poor baby, and no amount of therapy can cure the child once he or she is grown. They don't even want to think about the potential trauma to the baby if it's breech. Note: this assumption is total myth! The baby is not getting bumped on the head by the penis and this is no reason to stop having sex.

If your sex life has changed at some point in your pregnancy because your partner is afraid of hurting the baby, ask him if there is a position that would make him feel more safe. We always tell women to try to sleep on their left sides when they are pregnant. Maybe you could lie on your left side while he enters from behind. This puts you in a fancy position called *left lateral recumbent*, and perhaps by telling him this, he will feel more relaxed performing the deed.

As your body continues to expand, especially in the front, certain sexual positions may become extremely difficult to impossible. One that comes to mind as being almost impossible is the old standby, the missionary position. This is a great one for you because he has to do all of the work, and Lord knows you could use a break. The problem is, it might be hard for him to make good contact because of your big belly. Unless he can perform some sort of good teeter-totter impression and is able to bear all of his weight on his arms during the act, the missionary position may be somewhat dissatisfying during the last two months of the pregnancy. So, just like many of our politicians, you need to learn to change your position when the situation is uncomfortable. Let's briefly look at some of the positions one might consider.

The "woman-on-top" position brings the control back to you and can actually allow for a deeper penetration, as well as giving you the ability to do whatever you wish to bring about your orgasm. The true problem is that with control comes more work, and when you're thirty pounds heavier and sweating, who wants to do more work?

There is an old line by Steve Martin: "When she feels like a dog, we do it on the paper. When she feels like a cat, I have kitty litter." The "doggy-style" position (the man enters the woman from behind) is often fodder for comedians or shows like *Sex and the City*, but in reality, this can be a very comfortable way to have sex when you are extremely pregnant. I wouldn't try this method if you are one of the few women who has a small bladder, but if you really want to please your man, then this will be like a gift. The "cat position" is similar to missionary, but instead of resting on his elbows, the man places his hands under your arms and cups your shoulders.

Considering that this position increases frontal contact during a time when you are looking like Buddha, this position isn't recommended for very pregnant women.

The couple lying side by side as described above is comfortable for both partners and can be held for longer periods of time. This may be very beneficial for you if you are craving a longer sexual interlude. If you are merely trying to settle a debt, this will work too, but why not just use what you know will be the quickest for him?

In closing, we would like to remind you that there will soon be a seven- to eight-pound baby coming out of that vagina in a few months. If your partner is present at your delivery, he will see the ability of the vagina to stretch beyond what seems humanly possible. If he did not have a good sense of vaginal anatomy prior to the delivery, this may send him to the psychiatrist's office for treatment of post-traumatic stress disorder. Ease him in gently, and you yourself will feel comfortable with the size of your partner's penis. Remember, it's not the length of the rod, but the magic in the wand. No, that's not it. I'll just close with a slogan that I saw on a box of condoms for well-endowed men, "Because one size does not fit all." This was the best marketing slogan of all time. Who would buy the regular-sized condoms when those were so cleverly labeled?

If all else fails and you just can't seem to get him past the idea of having sex with his pregnant partner and he is becoming more aloof, remind him that there is no law against backrubs or just plain ol' spooning. Why does it always have to be about sex anyway? The important thing is to remain close, physically and emotionally. Touching in any loving way connects you physically, and usually some pretty pleasant emotions accompany the sensations. Relax and enjoy them.

8. I have been diagnosed as bipolar. Is it okay for me to be pregnant and take my medications?

Bipolar disorder (BD) is a fluctuation of mood between normal, depressive, and mania or hypomania. In order to be diagnosed with mania you would have to have elevated mood that inflates self-esteem, increased physical and sexual activity, and a display of poor judgment that potentially places you in less-than-ideal situations for more than one week. There have been studies on either side of the aisle when it comes to bipolar disorder in pregnancy. Some researchers have described an improvement in stability during pregnancy, while others have described no change at all.[4] The main issue with BD in pregnancy is maintaining good control and stability for the patient throughout the pregnancy. Along with psychotherapy, there may be more than one drug prescribed to help stabilize your mood if you have BD. Lithium is the standard choice for therapy and is considered safe, although it carries risks for mother and fetus. In the case of psychiatric diagnoses and treatment with medications, you should look at the side effects and decide if the risks are outweighed by the benefits. If the risks of a medicine are, say, 1 in 1,000, but if you rely on drugs or alcohol to solve your problems instead, then taking the medicine may be a better option.

9. Is it safe to take medication for my anxiety?

A certain amount of anxiety accompanies pregnancy. We think it is normal, for instance, for you to worry somewhat about delivery. Do you have a fear of labor and delivery? It has been reported that 10 to 20 percent of pregnant women have a fear of the delivery process. You may even have thought about asking for a cesarean delivery because of your fears. These are healthy concerns, yet they may cause excessive anxiety if you don't know what to expect. If your anxiety and worry start interfering with your daily life or are so consuming that you think of nothing else, then you should meet with a professional who can help you reduce these stressors.

Anxiety and fear have been shown to increase the risks of pre-eclampsia (a disorder of elevated blood pressure and possible maternal seizures).[5] As with most other times in life, severe anxiety will increase pain levels, which certainly is not desirable during labor. Women who have educated themselves about the labor process and who have good social support tend to have lower amounts of pain, and this may be due to decreased levels of anxiety. There are many studies showing that infants born to women with chronically elevated stress suffer from shortened gestation times and lower birth weights. There have also been multiple reported issues among children born to chronically stressed mothers. The main finding in a study of over 7,000 women with anxiety during pregnancy was that the risk doubled for hyperactivity in boys at four years of age.[6]

Obviously, some anxiety is normal. With our current economical crisis and the numbers of unemployed rising, it is doubtful that your life is not touched in some way by anxiety and stress. This stress becomes problematic when it prevents you from working or partaking in activities or attending functions you normally enjoy. Many patients with severe anxiety will be prescribed benzodiazepines (Valium, Xanax), and while these usually work well, they have a very substantial risk for abuse and addiction and so should not be used long term. Serotonin reuptake inhibitors like Prozac work well for those with anxiety and obsessive-compulsive disorder. We usually recommend medical therapies like Prozac when psychological therapies are either refused or not available. Again, a medication may fix an underlying chemical imbalance or mask the true depth of anxiety, but is it really getting at the root cause of the problem?

> I remember Gigi, a sweet, quiet nineteen-year-old patient in the second trimester of her first pregnancy. On one particular visit I noticed that she was constantly trying to clear her throat while I was talking. When she asked a question, she would rub her throat. It was almost as if she had something she wanted to say but was too afraid to ask. She had a normal exam, although she was a little behind on the weight gain, as she had only gained eight pounds over the last twenty weeks. As we discussed her eating habits, she continued to rub and clear her throat.
>
> I finally decided to ask her if there was something she wanted to ask me. She looked down at the floor and said no. I told her that I noticed she was rubbing her neck and clearing her throat like she had something stuck in there that she needed to get out. She looked up, and that was when the tears started to flow. She told me that she was very nervous about the fact that she worried that her husband was not going to be a good father because he had a problem with drugs and she did not want him to bring the drugs or the people with whom he associated into her house, especially after the baby was born. She had tried talking to him, but he always seemed distant or high and didn't want to talk about it with her. I asked her if she had a plan just in case she needed to leave him quickly, and she didn't, so we put together a plan and a place for her to go in case of emergency. I then asked her to bring her husband in to the next visit.

At the next visit I brought up the fact that she was worried about their abilities to parent with the current situation and that she was very scared and didn't know what to do. I asked him if he was willing to at least go to parenting classes with his wife, and he said that he was. I was hoping this would segue into getting him into a rehab program, but I didn't want to bite off more than he could chew. A few weeks later Gigi was back in the office with her husband and no longer had the nervous look or the scratchy throat. He had been going to classes with her, and she was feeling much more comfortable now that he was putting her and the baby first. He also said that being around other men changed the way he looked at being a father and he was ready to start on the road to recovery with his drug problem.

10. Hormones are strictly responsible for my mood swings.

This one is a myth. Just think about it. Too many other factors in life besides hormones affect our moods. As one group of researchers pointed out in 2008, social, psychological, behavioral, environmental, and biological forces are all at work within a person, influencing how he or she responds to major life events, as well as daily events. In addition, stress, family, and genetics can affect your pregnancy, your health, and your moods. Attributing mood swings to hormones would be clean and simple. Life, however, has far more texture woven into it, and all its threads influence how we act not only physically but emotionally. If you feel besieged by weighty emotional issues, finding outside help is beneficial not only to you but also to your baby.

> Stephanie was a seventeen-year-old struggling with a weight problem. For the last four or five years, she had been severely overweight and now, according to her body mass index (BMI), she was obese. Prior to becoming pregnant, she had started purposely vomiting after meals, a sign of the eating disorder called bulimia. When I first met her, she was depressed because of the pregnancy. She felt as though she would be gaining an excessive amount of weight. We discussed the issues surrounding her desires to lose weight and the healthier methods of weight loss. In many instances with obese patients it is perfectly safe to lose

weight during pregnancy or simply stay at your weight and not go up or down. Initially, we talked about the fact that she felt that eating made her feel better and that's why over the past five years she had gained sixty pounds. She was living on her own with her boyfriend, and they could afford dinner at the local fast-food restaurant but could not afford quality fruits and vegetables. Her bulimia had not yet affected her teeth or esophagus, but it was headed in that direction. I got her in to see a psychologist specializing in eating disorders. She also agreed to see a nutritionist who could help her make sound food choices. During her pregnancy she maintained a steady weight and had no complications as she dealt with her psychological trauma.

In this section of the book we have been focusing on early pregnancy myths and behaviors. We are now going to transition into the second and third trimesters to discuss myths surrounding gender, the delivery room, and superstitions about the baby. Just like your pregnancy, we are getting closer to the big day and need to discuss some of the myth-conceptions surrounding your upcoming delivery and your baby boy or girl.

Notes

1. H. A. Divan et al., "Prenatal and Postnatal Exposure to Cell Phone Use and Behavioral Problems in Children," *Epidemiology* 19, no. 4 (2008): 523.

2. Marie Osmond et al., *Behind the Smile: My Journey out of Postpartum Depression* (New York: Warner Books, 2001).

3. J. Evans, "Cohort Study of Depressed Mood during Pregnancy and after Childbirth," *British Medical Journal* 323 (2001): 257.

4. Ibid.; G. Faedda, L. Tondo, and R. Baldessarini, "Outcome after Rapid vs. Gradual Discontinuation of Lithium Treatment in Bipolar Disorders," *Archives of General Psychiatry* 50 (1993): 448.

5. T. Kurki, V. Hiielesma, and R. Raitalsalso, "Depression and Anxiety in Early Pregnancy and Risk for Preeclampsia," *Obstetrics & Gynecology* 95 (2000): 487.

6. T. G. O'Connor, J. Heron, and V. Glover, "Antenatal Anxiety Predicts Child Behavioral/Emotional Problems at 4 Years: Report from the AVON Longitudinal Study of Parents and Children," *British Journal of Psychiatry* 180 (2002): 502.

Section Four

Second and Third Trimester Myths

Chapter Seven

Gender Myths
Is It a Boy or a Girl?

S o you want to know the gender of your baby. Most people do, as soon as it is possible. You might even think that prospective parents who don't find out the gender of their baby before birth are weird. In our fast-paced world, control is everything. We have no patience for the unknown, a fact that is poignantly confirmed in the world of obstetrics. Most couples today will discern the sex of their child before birth via ultrasound. People want to know if they need to buy blue or pink, and they need to know if Pottery Barn has the right-colored bumper pads for that little boy or girl. But ultrasounds offer more information about the fetus than gender.

Between the sixteenth and twentieth weeks of gestation, the pregnant patient will have a level II ultrasound performed. This ultrasound measures the baby to pinpoint an accurate due date, but its main purpose is to complete an anatomic survey. Medically, we are looking at the circumference of the head and abdomen; the length of the long femur bone in the leg; imaging the brain, kidneys, and gastrointestinal tract; and looking at the chambers of the heart. What is foremost in the patient's and her family's minds, of course, is getting a look at the private parts. The technician performing the ultrasound can usually tell the expectant mother the gender of the baby at this stage. Anecdotally, we would say that about 95 percent of our patients elect to know the gender of their unborn child, although some surveys show the number to be only 65 to 80 percent. Although all mothers want to know that their baby is healthy and has all of the necessary functional parts, gender does seem to dominate the ultrasound experience.

This topic brings to mind a patient of mine and the issue between knowing or not knowing the gender of her baby.

K. B. was a twenty-eight-year-old female who was pregnant with her fifth child. Her previous pregnancies had produced four energetic boys, and she was eager to have a girl. I had the pleasure of delivering her fourth child, who was now thirteen months old, and joked that she could have a basketball team if she had another boy. Truth be told, she did not want to have another boy. Though this made her feel guilty, she openly discussed it with her husband and me. Her husband, an artillery sergeant, felt extremely proud to have fathered four boys. He now wanted another little guy to round out his basketball team. Their difference of opinions often caused a humorous scene in the office.

During her visit at eighteen weeks, K. B. had her ultrasound. Prior to the examination, the technician asked her if she wanted to know the sex of her baby. She stoically stated that she did not want to know the child's sex. This was a shock to both me and her husband. She didn't want to know about this little person until he or she came into the world because she wanted everyone to be happy rather than upset over the gender. Despite the protests of her husband, she simply stated that she had the final say since he wasn't the one carrying the baby. The older women in her family had convinced her that she was having another boy because of the way she was carrying the baby; they told her that she carried this pregnancy the same way she had carried the other four, and since they were all boys, well … Furthermore, the baby had a heart rate that was consistently under 140 beats per minute, and, according to her doting companions, this, too, meant she was having a boy. Furthermore, all of her nephews wanted her to pick them up, while the nieces did not seem to care as much. These three things were cause for the elder females in her family to declare, rather confidently, that K. B. would bear her fifth boy. Secretly, I think she was still holding out for that little bit of pink in her life.

During her ultrasound, I paid careful attention not to expose the baby's gender. Still with a strong desire to know, her husband asked if I would write the gender of the baby on a piece of paper and seal it in an envelope. He wanted this so he could potentially break the seal of the envelope if the anticipation got the better of him. His wife acquiesced to his request, and I wrote down the gender of the baby and sealed it.

The remainder of K. B.'s pregnancy transpired without complication. One evening, a labor and delivery nurse paged me, and we determined that K. B. was in labor. It was with excitement and anticipation that I entered the delivery room to share in the "surprise" moment. Right away I noticed the four young boys sitting between their aunt and grandmother on the sofa. Their ages spanned from ten to one, and their excitement was palpable. The little brothers had assembled some of their favorite clothes for the baby, as if they were dressing him in the team uniform. As the baby's head delivered, anticipation mounted, and with one final push K. B. delivered a beautiful baby girl. The cheers from the women in the room were countered with the hanging mouths of the little brethren on the couch. K. B.'s sister was so excited she hugged me as if I had something to do with the gender of her niece. I finished up, removed my protective gown, congratulated everyone, and turned for the door.

"Hey, Doc!" said K. B.'s husband.

I turned around to see him holding the unopened envelope from twenty weeks earlier.

"Wanna see if you were right?" He opened the envelope, pulled out a small piece of paper, and turned it around for all to see. In my handwriting, in capital letters, was the answer I had already known.

GIRL.

Myths about gender identification abound. Just like K. B.'s relatives, almost everyone seems to know at least one surefire way of identifying whether the unborn baby is a boy or a girl. The following are gender myths, old wives' tales, and superstitions that we frequently hear at the office. These myths and tales are often passed down through generations and are steeped in rich culture.

1. The manner in which the pregnant mother "carries" the baby gives a clue as to its gender.

The origin of this myth remains a mystery. How many women have heard that if you carry the baby high* then you're having a boy and if you carry the

---

*It's difficult to explain what "carrying high" means. Usually it means that your belly seems to protrude right from under your rib cage and immediately project outward. The woman carrying low on the other hand has a low, sloping belly that has more of a balled-up shape toward her pelvis.

baby in your pelvis it's a girl? Anatomically, the factors that affect how the uterus sits in the pelvis and abdomen are fetal size, maternal height, maternal weight, pelvic bony structure, position of the uterus, and the number of babies in the uterus. Assume that the baby is a boy. Would the fact that the baby has a penis affect the way in which the mother carries it? Many men might argue that the penis is the cause for the earth's rotation but are not as likely to think that a penis would influence the way a mother carries her baby.

Maternal height, on the other hand, affects the contour of the pregnant abdomen. A woman who is five feet tall may show signs of pregnancy* earlier than a woman who is six feet tall. A taller woman has more vertical space for the uterus, which may enable her to hide her pregnancy for a few more weeks. Maternal weight can also mask the signs of pregnancy. An obese woman, for instance, would not show signs of pregnancy until her later trimesters.

Pelvic bony structure is another factor. There are four maternal bony shapes of the pelvis. *Gynecoid* is the most common female pelvic shape, with a blunter, wider contour than a male pelvis. This pelvic shape is more likely to allow the fetus to drop lower in the pelvis, which means a woman may carry slightly lower. The *android* pelvis, also called male pelvis, is more heart-shaped and not conducive to a vaginal delivery. This pelvic shape may also cause the baby to stay higher in the pelvis and thus make a woman look as if she is carrying higher. The other two pelvic shapes are *platypelloid* and *anthropoid*. The platypelloid is an oval from side to side, and the anthropoid is oval from front to back; both of these shapes make it more difficult for the baby's head to drop into the pelvis.

I had just finished seeing a patient of mine who was about twenty-eight weeks pregnant and had brought her Mexican grandmother in with her to hear the fetus's heart beat. She and her grandmother were very pleasant people, and as we finished her appointment, we continued to talk as I walked them to the front desk. I was pregnant as well, at that time, and about as far along as this patient was. They both asked me if I knew what the sex of my baby was. I explained that I did not, and that I wanted it to be a surprise. The grandmother was very curious about this and felt the need to investigate further. She asked me to turn around. I asked her, "You

---

*These are the physical signs like the bulge in your belly and walking with a different gait. A woman whose torso is shorter than the uterus will fill the pelvis and torso in a quicker fashion and she will have a bigger belly faster than a woman with a longer torso.

mean turn my back to you?" She said yes. So I did. She then replied, "Well, you're having a boy." I laughed nervously, wondering why she would think that and not sure that I really wanted to know. But I did ask, "What makes you say that?" She then replied, "Well, my dear, I saw you before when you weren't pregnant, and your butt wasn't that big." In the end (no pun intended), we did have a boy, so this patient's mother was correct. Of course she had a 50-50 chance of guessing correctly.

2. If the fetal heart rate is below 140 beats per minute, it's a boy; if it's above 140, it's a girl.

From ten weeks until delivery, a routine doctor's visit includes listening to the fetal heart rate with a Doppler device.* Many patients ask us whether or not the heart rate of the baby can determine its gender. Although we've heard it reversed occasionally, it seems to be widely accepted by most patients that a heart rate above 140 is most likely to be a girl. This myth crosses all cultures and age groups. No one seems to know where it came from. In fact, in our research, few theories even exist.

Studies, however, show no significant difference between a male and a female heart rate, at least statistically speaking.[1] The normal heart rate for a fetus is anywhere from 120 to 160 beats per minute. The heart rate will fluctuate from beat to beat and demonstrates what is called fetal heart rate variability. The developing fetal brain is controlled by the sympathetic nervous system (the fight-or-flight response) and the parasympathetic (relaxation) system. As the brain develops, these two systems engage in a power struggle. The heart rate speeds up when stimulated by the sympathetic system and slows down when controlled by the parasympathetic response. So, depending on the arousal of the fetus, the heart rate can be 130 on one day, 110 the next, and 150 the next. We usually listen to the fetal heart rate for about ten to thirty seconds at a time. If the baby is awake and moving, the heart rate may be higher than if it is sleeping.

We can extrapolate this theory. Men and women, boys and girls do not

---

*Dopplers work on the principle of listening to reflections of small, high-frequency sound waves (ultrasound). These ultrasound waves are generated by microscopic vibrations of piezoelectric crystals. When the waves are reflected from moving objects, such as a fetal heart, the frequency changes slightly. It is this change that is analyzed by the electronics of the Doppler and converted into an audible sound or a digital display of the heart rate.

have different heart rates based on gender. The heart rate in a healthy individual is a response to external stimuli and not necessarily caused by the gender of the individual.

3. If the pregnant woman craves spicy or tart foods, then she is having a boy.

Cravings in pregnancy are satirized in movies, TV shows, and commercials. The classic parody shows a pregnant woman waking her husband in the middle of the night to go out and buy pickles and ice cream. Cravings can be complicated, multidimensional, and unique to every individual, but hormones and nutritional imbalances certainly play a role.

We are often asked if craving spicy foods means that a boy is on the way. As we currently practice in Tucson, Arizona, where Mexican food is commonplace, you would think that, if this were the case, we would have a preponderance of male births. Women (and men) tend to crave foods that they enjoy: I like it, so I eat it. During pregnancy, the placenta secretes high levels of progesterone, a hormone that stimulates the appetite center in the brain. This stimulation can trigger a craving for foods that one may already find appealing.

Pica (mentioned previously) is defined as an abnormal craving that is due to anemia (usually brought on by iron deficiency), which is very common in pregnancy. Such cravings are not a common manifestation of anemia. A classic example of pica is the woman who has an uncontrollable desire to consume unusual items like dirt or soap. A more unusual example is one mentioned earlier, that of the patient who was strongly attracted to the smell of tire rubber. She understood that consuming tires was not a part of the pregnancy plan, but nonetheless she had a strong desire to chew on a tire. Thankfully, this woman did not have this same urge during her next pregnancy.

"Girls are made of sugar and spice and everything nice; boys are made from snakes and snails and puppy dog tails." This rather sexist nursery rhyme depicts males as harsh and caustic and females as nurturing and sweet. Perhaps this rhyme has helped perpetuate the myth that a pregnant woman who craves spicy food is destined to deliver a boy.*

---

*We understand that this only applies to cultures in which boys and men are considered more harsh and caustic. In cultures or subcultures where the woman might be the abrasive or tougher individual, this myth might be potentially reversed.

3a. Eating peppers or hot spices during pregnancy will cause my baby to suffer from colic.

We have included this dietary myth as a subset of the preceding question, since it belongs in the spicy foods category. Again, many people enjoy spicy foods; many babies are born with colic. Are the two related?

If your baby cries around the same time every day and is inconsolable, your baby may have colic. Colic is traditionally defined as crying for more than three hours a day, three days a week, for more than three weeks. Colic affects 25 percent of babies.[2] Fortunately, 90 percent of these cases resolve themselves by the time the child reaches nine months of age.*

It's currently not known what causes colic, but women who smoke during pregnancy or after delivery give birth to infants with twice the rate of colic.[3] Colic doesn't seem to occur any more frequently in females than in males, and it hasn't been shown to be related to the diet of a mother who breastfeeds.

You and your baby have completely separate dietary tracts. The fetus does receive its nutrition from you, but not in the form of solid food. Rather, the fetus receives nutrition across the placenta in the form of nutrients within the blood supply it shares with the mother. Examples of these nutrients are protein, fat, and carbohydrates. When you eat a chili pepper, it's broken down into its various nutrients, one of which is called capsaicin, an antioxidant. All peppers, in fact, contain antioxidants, which are actually good for both you and your baby. Antioxidants play many roles, including combating free radicals, which are linked to causing cancer.

We have never had a colicky child, and our hearts go out to those parents who have comforted their children through this process. The fear of having a baby with colic is potentially so strong that this myth may have evolved in an attempt to eliminate this unfortunate but temporary problem.

---

*Researchers are not certain why this occurs.

4. **If you crack a raw egg on the mother's belly,
   the side to which it slides predicts the gender
   of the baby. If the egg slides to the mother's right,
   it is a boy, and if it slides to the left, it is a girl.**

Other than being messy, this superstition offers no obvious merit. The shape of the mother's belly and point where the yolk of the egg lands will determine the direction the egg slides. What does it mean if the egg stays on the belly and doesn't slide? When we investigated the meaning and purpose of this myth, we discovered the egg's symbolism. The Mystical World Egg, for instance, embodies the entire universe in its embryo. In the Orient, the egg represents creation and contains heaven and hell in the two halves of the shell. The egg can also symbolize the bisexual potential of the embryo and its ability to develop into a male or a female. Ancient Egyptians portrayed the world egg as being similar to the egg inside a woman's uterus.

As you can probably imagine, there have been no studies to confirm or invalidate the egg-cracking gender test. But it remains one of our favorites due to the symbolism and unique nature of the myth.

5. **If you tie the pregnant woman's wedding band
   to a chain and dangle it over her belly, the direction
   of the spin will tell the gender of the baby.**

If you dangle a wedding band or other item, like a safety pin, from a chain, it will rotate in a particular direction. This happens whether or not it is dangled over a pregnant woman or an obese man. In looking into this myth, we have not been able to discern which direction of spin is considered to be male or female. The general belief seems to be that a clockwise spin indicates a male and a counterclockwise spin, a female. It's been shown that the unconscious desires of the individual holding the chain can cause a particular rotation, because that person unwittingly makes certain movements. Therefore, if the person holding the chain knows that clockwise means boy, and he or she would like a boy, there is a greater likelihood that the ring will spin in a clockwise manner.

In myths or superstitions that involve a right and a left spin or side, the male designation is usually to the right and the female to the left.

According to the lore, right-handedness means clever or skillful, while left-handedness is associated with being witchlike or diabolical.[4] Throughout history the left side has been associated with the feminine. Ancient Greeks would tattoo themselves with a male symbol on the right and a female symbol on the left. During medieval times, popular belief held that a boy came from the right testicle and a girl from the left.[5] Right-handed masculinity also appears in Christianity with Christ being seated at the right hand of the Father.

Another interesting aspect of this myth involves the wedding ring. For centuries, people believed that a vein extended from the ring finger of a woman's left hand directly to her heart.[6] Therefore, if a dangled ring rotates to the left, this shows a connection to the female side and indicates that the infant is a girl.

Going back to the medieval thought that boys came from the right testicle, men who wanted a boy would cut off their left testicle. Today, we have two less drastic approaches to selecting gender. One method, called MicroSort, reportedly can increase the chances of having a girl by 90 percent. This method, however, can only be used in conjunction with artificial insemination or in vitro fertilization, which entails obtaining eggs from the mother surgically, fertilizing the egg with the sperm in the lab, and eventually re-implanting the eggs in the mother's reproductive tract. The MicroSort technology utilizes the scientific data that "boy" sperm weigh less than "girl" sperm. The reason that "boy" sperm are lighter is because they have a Y-chromosome, which contains less DNA, or data. The "girl" sperm contains an "X" chromosome that contains a large portion of DNA. So this weight factor plays a role in how the fertilization process is accomplished.

The Shettles method is much less expensive and easier to utilize, since it doesn't require a laboratory or surgery. It merely relies on the timing of sexual intercourse. The same principle applies: "boy" sperm are lighter and thereby faster and more fragile than "girl" sperm. In the Shettles method, if you want to have a boy, you have sex at the exact time of ovulation, so that the fastest "boy" sperm arrive to the egg first. If you want to have a girl, you have intercourse about two and a half to three days before ovulation, because the "girl" sperm can live longer and can take their time navigating the reproductive tract. The data on the Shettles method are limited. One study actually showed that the timing of intercourse has no bearing on the sex of the baby.[7]

6. The Chinese Birth Calendar is the test most predictive of fetal gender.

The Chinese Birth Calendar is a chart that was supposedly discovered approximately seven hundred years ago in Beijing and currently resides at the Beijing Institute of Science. This calendar is said to predict the fetus's gender by factoring together maternal age and the month in which the mother conceived. We first heard of this chart/calendar from our sister-in-law, who explained to us that she had heard that the calendar accurately predicts gender 99 percent of the time. This obviously piqued our interest. Whenever you hear that something is 99 percent accurate, you pay attention.

Basically, the chart consists of two axes. The vertical axis plots the age of the mother at conception, while the horizontal axis plots the month in which the pregnancy was conceived. Lines are drawn on the chart, and the point at which the lines intersect is where you find the gender of the fetus.

We want the reader to know that, just for fun, we went through a small sample of ten charts in our office of women who had delivered with us. We reviewed the ultrasound determination of fetal gender along with the actual gender determined at the time of birth, and these were compared to the Chinese calendar prediction. We discovered that the Chinese calendar method was correct in nine out of the ten cases.

In further analyzing this method of gender prediction, there are some remarkable generalizations that can be made. According to the calendar, if a woman conceives when she is eighteen years of age, she has an 80 percent chance of having a girl. If she conceives when she is twenty-one, she has a 90 percent chance of having a girl. We could not think of any medical reason or study that demonstrated why a woman would have a girl 90 percent of the time during one calendar year of her life and not another. A simple look at the delivery log book at our labor and delivery center did not demonstrate this effect.

Two variables in the calendar could be cause for error. The first is the actual month of conception. Most due dates are determined by the woman's first day of her last menstrual period. In reality, conception doesn't occur until at least two weeks after the last menstrual period. Pregnancy begins once the sperm and the egg meet in the fallopian tube, and that only occurs after ovulation, which is usually about two weeks after the first day of the last menstrual period. For example, if your last menstrual period was

Month of Conception

Age	Jan	Feb	Mar	Apr	May	Jun	Jul	Aug	Sep	Oct	Nov	Dec
18	F	M	F	M	M	M	M	M	M	M	M	M
19	M	F	M	F	F	M	M	F	M	M	F	F
20	F	M	F	M	M	M	M	M	M	F	M	M
21	M	F	F	F	F	F	F	F	F	F	F	F
22	F	M	M	F	M	F	F	M	F	F	F	F
23	M	M	M	F	M	M	F	F	F	M	M	F
24	M	F	F	M	M	F	M	F	M	M	F	M
25	F	M	F	M	F	M	F	M	F	M	M	M
26	M	M	M	M	M	F	M	F	F	M	F	F
27	F	F	M	M	F	M	F	F	M	F	M	M
28	M	M	M	F	F	M	F	M	F	M	F	M
29	F	M	F	F	M	F	M	M	F	M	F	F
30	M	M	F	M	F	M	M	M	M	M	M	M
31	M	M	M	M	F	F	M	F	M	F	F	F
32	M	F	F	M	F	M	M	F	M	M	F	M
33	F	M	M	F	F	M	F	M	F	M	M	F
34	M	M	F	F	M	F	M	M	F	M	F	F
35	M	F	M	F	M	F	M	F	M	M	F	M
36	M	F	M	M	M	F	M	M	F	F	F	F
37	F	F	M	F	F	F	M	F	F	M	M	M
38	M	M	F	F	M	F	F	M	F	F	M	F
39	F	F	M	F	F	F	M	F	M	M	F	M
40	M	M	M	F	M	F	M	F	M	F	F	M
41	F	F	M	F	M	M	F	F	M	F	M	F
42	M	F	F	M	M	M	M	M	F	M	F	M
43	F	M	F	F	M	M	M	F	F	F	M	M
44	M	F	F	F	M	F	M	M	F	M	F	M
45	F	M	F	M	F	F	M	F	M	F	M	F

The Chinese Birth Calendar. Try it out and
see if it is accurate for your child's gender.

October 24, you likely became pregnant at or around November 7. So in this case, conception occurred in November, not October.

The second variable that gives cause for error pertains to the mother's age. According to the calendar, the age used is the mother's age at the time she delivers. The only way to know that is to wait until the delivery, since there are two weeks both before and after the actual due date that are factors in a full-term pregnancy, anywhere from thirty-eight to forty-two weeks.

There is also the possibility of having a preterm, or premature baby, which obviously wouldn't be predictable until after delivery either and therefore not of much use for those wanting to know gender prior to delivery.

7. Ultrasound is 100 percent predictive of the baby's gender.

An ultrasound is performed in the second trimester to determine the size and anatomy of your baby and to confirm the correct due date for the pregnancy, along with giving the parents reassurance that all is well. Again, we have to say that most couples are very concerned with the gender of the baby at the time of this ultrasound. Obviously, the couple wants a healthy baby, but is it a healthy baby boy or girl? In this age where immediate gratification is the norm, we no longer have to wait until delivery to discover the sex of the baby. There is a small percentage of couples, like us, that did not choose to know the gender of their children until they were born. We will have to go on record stating that Shawn wanted to know and Katie did not, and thus with the 51 percent veto power of the pregnant mother, we did not know the gender until birth.

Wanting to know the gender of our baby became an obsession to the point where I asked my wife daily if I could look at the ultrasound machine in the office, but to no avail. What made things worse for me were the throngs of friends and family asking, and their looks of total disbelief. "You mean you guys don't know what you are having? What, don't you know how to do an ultrasound?" In the end, I discovered that, as the father, as well as the obstetrician, it is truly exciting to have *and* deliver a baby whose gender is unknown.

So what is the success rate of ultrasound in gender prediction? It really depends on the gestational age of the infant when the scan is performed and the skill of the technician performing the ultrasound. In the early second trimester, around fourteen to fifteen weeks, the sex of the fetus can be difficult to visualize because the penis and the clitoris have a similar developmental structure. An ultrasound done around eighteen to twenty weeks of gestation has a higher predictive value for gender. In fact, studies have shown that sex can be determined 100 percent of the time if the ultrasound is done after twenty weeks in at least one or two exams. In a review of multiple studies, the accuracy was shown to be 97 percent.[8]

Ultrasound reports from outside facilities not associated with our birthing clinic almost never state the gender of the baby. Ultrasound centers commonly discourage their technicians from going on record with the gender of the fetus for fear of retribution if they are wrong. We have yet to hear of a lawsuit against someone for telling the parents that the gender of the baby was different than expected, but things happen. So if ultrasound can be wrong and the Chinese calendar is questionable, what can you do if you want to know the sex of your baby? The answer in most cases: wait and see.

The only other option is amniocentesis, a test in which a needle is placed through the abdominal wall and into the uterus and used to draw a small bit of amniotic fluid, which is sent to a lab. A chromosomal analysis of the fetus is done, which determines the sex of the baby. This test is normally performed for women over age thirty-five or those concerned about a possible chromosomal defect. The risk of the amniotic membranes rupturing during or after the procedure is about one in two hundred. Because such a rupture can cause life-threatening issues for the baby, this test is inappropriate for gender determination. Currently, the test is only offered by obstetricians and maternal-fetal medicine specialists who have a clearly documented medical reason for performing it.

8. Mixing the mother's urine with crystal Drāno will tell you the gender based on a color change in the urine when the two are mixed.

Many years ago, we were listening to a morning talk show in the Oklahoma City area that solicited women who were willing to share stories about how they tested for the gender of their babies. The radio channel gathered five methods of gender prediction from their listening audience, then set out to determine which method was the most accurate. It's difficult to remember which methods were pitted against each other, but the test that was deemed most reliable entailed mixing crystal Drāno with urine.

Drāno, manufactured by SC Johnson & Sons, is a product used for cleaning household drains. Developed by a chemist, it contains sodium hydroxide, sodium nitrate, sodium chloride, and aluminum. A multitude of Web sites suggest a variety of methods for mixing the Drāno with urine. Once the urine and Drāno are mixed, you can tell the gender of your baby based on the color of the mixture. Supposedly, if the mixture turns brown, black, or dark blue, your baby is a boy. If the mixture is clear, green, or light blue, you can expect a girl. We're not sure where this test originated or who had the time to conjure it, but Drāno is very caustic and the fumes created can cause injury. This test should be relegated to the archives and for early morning radio fodder. We implore you not to even think about trying it.

9. A European tradition claims that in order to determine the gender of your baby, an older woman, preferably your mother, should throw salt on your hair when you're not expecting it. If you move your hand to your forehead first, you will have a boy; if you move your hand to your chin first, you will have a girl.

You're an unsuspecting victim at the annual Fourth of July picnic. Your mother sneaks up behind you and throws a dash of salt into your hair. For the next minutes to hours, all eyes are on you to see if you touch your chin or your forehead first. What happens if you have an itch on your behind?

Enough said.

10. If the baby tightens up in your stomach like a ball, then you're having a boy.

This, in fact, is quite "true." The reason we put that in quotations is because this statement was posted on an online pregnancy forum. The participant who made the comment felt that, although many of the items discussed previously were false, this particular myth was most definitely true. It is not.

When you feel your uterus contracting or "balling up" in your stomach, you are more than likely experiencing a contraction. Uterine contractions experienced on and off during the second and third trimesters are called Braxton-Hicks contractions* and are typically more

---

*Braxton-Hicks contractions are different from regular labor contractions because they do not occur in any kind of pattern. With Braxton-Hicks contractions, you may contract once or twice an hour, but the next hour you may have none or you might have one in the next two hours and then nothing for the rest of the day. If the contractions begin to organize into a pattern, you should call your physician.

irritating than preterm or term labor patterns. The uterine contractions do not dictate the gender of your baby.

11. If other babies or toddlers approach an expectant mother, then she will have a baby of that gender. If boy toddlers want her to hold them more than girls, then she must be having a boy, and vice versa.

In order to predict gender in this way, you would have to keep a running tally of the percentages of boys versus girls who want pregnant women to hold them. Nine months is a long time. Does this pertain to the entire pregnancy or just certain trimesters? The way children react to pregnancies will vary greatly. If the woman happens to have candy in her hand, she may attract every toddler around—which means she might be having sextuplets.

We are not aware of any specific pheromones or chemicals given off by a pregnant woman carrying a particularly engendered baby. You can shelve this one next to the Drāno bottle.

12. Faster hair growth on your legs means you will have a boy.

We have to believe that this myth came to exist because men have more hair on their legs than women...in most cases. Rest assured that hair has nothing to do with the baby's gender. But this myth does give us the opportunity to discuss hair growth during pregnancy.

Many women notice that the hair on their heads is thicker during pregnancy. These same women find their hair falling out in clumps during the postpartum period. Hair growth usually returns to its normal cycle within about six months after delivery. In a normal cycle, each hair grows about a half inch per month. There are three stages of hair growth, and all hair follicles alternate between these three phases: growth, involution, and resting. At any given time about 10 percent of your hair is in the resting phase. During pregnancy, due to the changes in levels of different hormones in your bloodstream, more of your hair follicles get "stuck" in the resting phase for a longer duration. This causes less hair to fall out while you are pregnant, thus causing it to look fuller. In other words, hair that you would normally have lost during pregnancy tends to stay put, making it seem like you actually have more hair. After delivery, this resting phase shortens, giving the impression that you are losing your hair when in reality you are losing the hair that would have come out normally if you were not pregnant. Some women will develop more hair on the chin, upper lip, cheeks, arms, and legs during pregnancy. You may also notice new hair on your breasts, belly, and back. This is due to an increased production of pregnancy hormones and cortisol.* The effect will also seem more pronounced in women with darker hair.

13. The missionary position makes boys.

We have already discussed that both the speed and the weight of the sperm have a potential to determine the sex of the baby, but what about the position in which the pregnancy was conceived? There is no medical evidence to suggest that the missionary ("man-on-top") position is more likely to produce a boy baby, other than various presumptions made regarding the facts about male sperm. Actually, there is a basic lack of medical evidence for this myth because no one has designed a reliable test to prove this claim. No doubt it has something to do with the precarious nature of attempting to make such a test reproducible and respectable. Need we say more?

14. You must be having a boy because your husband has only brothers.

Gender does not run in a family. At some point, the family tree has to include at least a few branches of women or else the tree would look more like a family twig. Because women are chromosomally XX, a woman can donate only an X chromosome to her fetus; in other words, women can only beget women. Men, on the other hand, can donate an X or a Y chromosome,

---

*Cortisol is a steroid hormone produced by the adrenal cortex, which mediates various metabolic processes, has anti-inflammatory and immunosuppressive properties, and whose levels in the blood may become elevated in response to physical or psychological stress.

and thus, depending on which one they donate, the baby will be a boy or a girl. We are not aware of any genetic predisposition that would result in a male with only Y chromosome–loaded sperm. This would seem counter-intuitive to the propagation of our species. The species needs women to be in abundant supply since they are the ones who carry the pregnancy.

15. If you already have two boys or two girls, then your next baby will be the same sex.

Again, this theory pays undo credence to the fact that sperm from the male determines the sex of the baby. For the most part, whether he donates a Y chromosome or an X chromosome is out of his control. We have heard of this myth stating the third child will be the same gender as the last two, but it does not seem to apply to women having their second, fourth, or fifth child. Is there magic to the number three?

> An equilateral triangle has three equal sides.
> A human ear has three semicircular canals.
> The psyche has three parts (id, ego, superego).
> Noah had three sons.
> Plato split the soul into three parts.
> The three R's (Reading, wRiting, aRithmetic).
> Bad luck comes in threes.
> Three children outnumber their parents.

16. If my baby is born on an odd day, it will be a boy.

It may seem strange, but when considering the esoteric belief in the power of numbers, or numerology, there is a distinction given to odd numbers. Odd numbers are said to correspond to the right side of the brain and to relate to adventure, stress, and the ability to work within one's path by managing stress and going with the flow. In a patriarchal society these would seem to be male traits and might be the reason for this myth of males being born on odd days. In a society ruled by matriarchs, it may be that the word "odd" simply refers to the fact that men are considered odd. This is said in jest, but it is food for thought. Again, we have disproved this claim easily just by looking at the delivery log at our labor and delivery center.

17. When a pregnant woman is asked to show her hands, if she shows them palms up, it is a girl, palms down, it's a boy.

This can be looked at in a number of ways. In his discussion on body language, Adam Eason describes people as tending to behave more honestly when they display their open palms to others. Are girls more honest than boys? Not likely, and certainly very difficult to prove. In ancient times the palm-up gesture showed that you were not holding any weapons in a display of trust. Eason also describes that the palm facing up is a submissive and nonthreatening gesture, whereas the palm-down gesture projects authority. Perhaps this old wives' tale is propagated simply because it relates to a male-dominated, premodern society.

18. If you prefer lying on your left side, you are having a girl.

The left side, in historical reference, is often related to the feminine. Why do healthcare providers instruct pregnant women to lie on their left sides? Here is a medical explanation: The largest vein in the body is called the vena cava. This blood vessel drains the lower extremities and brings blood flow back to the heart, which then pumps the blood through the lungs for oxygenation. The vena cava is slightly to the right of midline in the human body. When the enlarged pregnant uterus is pressing on the vena cava, it can decrease the blood flow returning to the heart and thus decrease the amount of blood pumping back out to the placenta and the fetus. If the pregnant woman lies on her left side, the pressure is theoretically released from the vena cava, thus maintaining regular blood flow. Having to lie on one's left side can cause great distress in pregnant women who may prefer to sleep on their stomachs but no longer can because of discomfort. Constantly lying on the left side can result in back pain, and many women are afraid to sleep on their backs. But tucking a small pillow under the right hip and lower back is often enough of a tilt to restore ample blood flow without having to lie fully on one's left side. Ultimately, however, lying on one's left side is not a gender predictor and definitely not worth losing sleep over—especially in a state that is already designed for insomnia.

19. If you crave the heels from a loaf of bread, you are having a boy.

We have seen this claim on several Web sites, always in the form of a question. We have yet to find an answer. It is difficult to find anything to say about this one, although we are somewhat curious to know how this adage would translate to cultures that use flatbreads. Typically, the heel from a loaf of bread is considered the crusty, hard piece that many people discard. For some, especially according to Irish tales, the heel is considered the best piece of the loaf. How this activity could determine a baby's gender escapes us completely.

20. Eat a clove of garlic and if the smell is discernable from your skin, you are having a boy.

Much like myth number 3 above, this may be a remnant of the nursery rhyme about the nature of boys. It seems that boys are associated with things repugnant. Any person eating a large quantity of garlic would have halitosis, and her sweat and skin oils would smell like garlic. According to the Christian Bible, when Satan left the Garden of Eden, garlic grew from his left footprint. However, in ancient times, garlic did not have the smelly disposition it has today. It was used for multiple medicinal purposes and was held in high esteem. In European myth, garlic was used for protection. Hindus feel that garlic stimulates the body and provokes the desires. Because it would be difficult to eat a raw clove of garlic, this myth more than likely came from a culture familiar with the taste and power of this medicinal plant.

So, why do you want to know the gender of your baby? Is it because you want to meet him or her (at least in your mind) sooner? Such knowledge definitely makes the baby shower easier, because you can tell your friends whether to buy pink or blue. Wanting to know the gender of our baby demonstrates our need to control our surroundings. It is rare for a couple to go through the whole pregnancy and not know whether they are having a boy or a girl. We would venture to say that, in our practice, we've seen only a few couples each year who don't want to know the sex of their baby.

Remember that Shawn wanted to know the birth of our first baby, but Katie did not. Today Shawn says that, although it was difficult waiting all those months, the day of the delivery—as the baby was coming out and nobody in the room knew whether it would be a boy or a girl—was probably one of the most exciting times he has ever experienced.

Notes

1. D. S. McKenna et al., "Gender Related Differences in Fetal Heart Rate during First Trimester," *Fetal Diagnosis and Therapy* 21, no. 1 (2006): 144.

2. http://www.mayoclinic.com/health/colic/DS00058 (accessed January 2, 2009).

3. C. Sondergaard et al., "Smoking during Pregnancy and Infantile Colic," *Pediatrics* 108 (2001): 342.

4. B. Walker, *The Women's Encyclopedia of Myths and Secrets* (San Francisco: Harper, 1983).

5. http://www.thetech.org/genetics/ask.php?id=76 (accessed January 10, 2009).

6. http://www.unexplainedstuff.com/Superstitions-Strange-Customs -Taboos-and-Urban-Legends/Strange-Customs-and-Taboos-Courtship-and -marriage.html (accessed January 2, 2009).

7. A. J. Wilcox, C. R. Weinberg, and D. D. Baird, "Timing of Sexual Intercourse in Relation to Ovulation: Effect on the Probability of Conception/Survival of Pregnancy and Sex of the Baby," *New England Journal of Medicine* 333, no. 32 (1995): 1511.

8. B. R. Elajalde, M. M. Elajalde, and T. Heitman, "Visualization of the Fetal Genitalia by Ultrasonography, a Review of the Literature and Analysis of Its Accuracy and Ethical Implications," *Journal of Ultrasound in Medicine* 12, no. 4 (1985): 633.

Chapter Eight

Preterm Labor and Delivery Myths
Fashionably Early

∽⌒∽

I t's the thirty-eighth week of your pregnancy and boy, oh, boy (or girl, oh, girl), are you ready to bring this baby into the world. Of course, it's best for all involved if the baby arrives as close as possible to the fortieth week, because all organ systems will be fully developed, but if you do go into labor at this point, it will be considered a full-term labor. There will be no need to put the brakes on your contractions. If contractions begin prior to this week, however, then your labor is considered to be preterm labor.

If you are between your twentieth and thirty-seventh week of pregnancy and you start experiencing contractions more than every fifteen minutes or if you're leaking water, you should make a beeline to your hospital's labor and delivery unit. No pregnant woman wants to go into premature labor, because her baby will not be fully developed and will face at least temporary health challenges. Almost everyone knows someone who delivered early.

Preterm labor is a subject infiltrated by misinformation and myths. While it's frightening to go into labor early, knowing the facts about what triggers it and how it is handled medically can quell fears. Knowledge is a good thing. So let's step into the world of preterm labor and separate fact from fiction.

Before we begin differentiating between preterm labor myths and truths, we need to provide a bit of background. The definition of preterm labor is similar to that of regular labor, with one exception. Preterm labor occurs between weeks twenty and thirty-seven of pregnancy, whereas full-term labor occurs from weeks thirty-seven to forty-two. Even if you go into labor at thirty-six weeks and six days, you are considered to be in preterm labor.

In the United States, about 12 to 13 percent of pregnancies end up in preterm labor, typically called premature labor. The concern for the baby is that the major organ systems don't fully develop until between thirty-two and thirty-seven weeks. Though premature babies born between twenty-four and thirty-seven weeks can survive, these *preemies* may have long-term health challenges including breathing and digestive difficulties, learning disabilities, and developmental problems.

1. If I go into preterm labor, I can count on treatments to stop it.

This statement is a myth. No medication currently on the market has been shown to completely stop preterm labor. However, there are treatments to slow or temporarily halt contractions that give physicians more time to help the baby mature. Should you go into preterm labor, here are some common pharmaceuticals your healthcare provider might give you:

- **Magnesium sulfate.** Used since the 1970s to arrest labor, magnesium sulfate has an established track record. Since physicians know its side effects and how best to administer it, they often turn to it as a first-line treatment. Scientists do not know exactly how it works in the body, though they speculate that it reduces the calcium in muscle cells required for contraction. The Cochrane Collaboration, a group of researchers that routinely evaluates the current medical research, found that using magnesium sulfate during the first forty-eight hours of preterm labor did not significantly decrease preterm birthrate. It did, however, slow preterm uterine contractions in some women. If preterm labor can be halted, even for up to a week, steroids can be administered to hasten the baby's development. When steroids are administered after forty-eight hours of premature labor, they improve the baby's lung function, cut the rate of lung disease in half, and reduce the baby's risk of dying by 40 percent.

Common side effects of magnesium sulfate for the mother include flushing, nausea, headache, drowsiness, and blurred vision. All are temporary. The fetus also may experience side effects related to respiratory and motor functions. Women on magnesium sulfate, as well as any other preterm labor medications, are carefully monitored.

Maria, a twenty-nine-year-old, was pregnant for the third time. She had one previous pregnancy delivered after her due date and one that ended in miscarriage. She had been problem free this time, until her thirtieth week. Maria worked long hours as a wait-ress at a local diner and hefted great weights overhead as she delivered food. Because she weighed only one hundred and thirty pounds, I used to joke that she was like an ant, capable of carrying many times her body weight. One day she called my medical assis-tant at the office and said that she was experiencing cramps at work, but they decreased a little if she sat down or rested. We instructed her to go home, drink plenty of fluids, rest, and call us back if the cramping exceeded every fifteen minutes or grew stronger. She called back a few hours later and said that the con-tractions were closer and they were beginning to hurt.

Maria went to the hospital, where monitors confirmed that she was in preterm labor. Her uterine contractions were spaced five to ten minutes apart, and her cervix had dilated to three cen-timeters (about the diameter when you place middle and index fingers together to form a circle). Prior to checking her cervix, the nurse had swabbed it to test for a chemical called fetal fibronectin (we will discuss this later in this chapter). Then she started intra-venous fluids.

Because the fluids did not stop Maria's contractions, we started her on magnesium sulfate in an attempt to at least slow down the labor so that we could administer antibiotics and betamethasone* (a corticosteroid). The antibiotic was given to protect the baby from group B streptococcus (GBS). GBS resides on the skin in over 30 percent of the population and is considered

---

*Betamethasone dipropionate is a synthetic glucocorticoid that is used topically on the skin. (The naturally occurring glucocorticoid is cortisol or hydrocortisone, which is produced by the adrenal gland.) Glucocorticoids have potent anti-inflammatory actions and also suppress the immune response.

a normal skin flora. In newborns, however, it is the leading cause of meningitis and pneumonia. The betamethasone was administered to speed up fetal lung maturity; it can also protect the brain from bleeding during the birthing process.

After the administration of magnesium sulfate, antibiotics, and steroids, Maria's contractions slowed and eventually stopped for three days. Then, they broke through again, regardless of our efforts. Maria went into labor again and had to be transferred to a facility that could care for a thirty-week-old baby. She delivered the day after we sent her to University Medical Center at the University of Arizona. Her baby did very well but had to spend three weeks in the neonatal nursery before he was allowed to go home.

Maria's story is fairly typical of a woman in preterm labor. When labor begins earlier, say, between twenty-four and twenty-eight weeks, physicians may try different methods besides magnesium sulfate to slow contractions. For those women closer to thirty-six weeks, doctors may do nothing at all, since the baby will more than likely do fine if he or she is born this far into the pregnancy.

- **Calcium channel blockers.** These medications are routinely used to treat high blood pressure, chest pain, and irregular heart rates. Nifedipine* is the name of the calcium channel blocker most specific to the uterus. Since fetal side effects are low, nifedipine is being used more frequently. Maternal side effects are few but bothersome, headache and low blood pressure being the most common. If you're taking nifedipine, make sure you stay well hydrated. The number of preterm births within seven days of treatment and before thirty-four weeks gestation were significantly reduced when this medication was used.[2]
- **Cyclooxygenase inhibitors.** Cyclooxygenase inhibitors block a chemical called prostaglandin, which is used to induce labor. The name of the cyclooxygenase inhibitor targeted to preterm labor is indomethacin. The Cochrane Collaboration concluded that indomethacin reduced the rate of preterm birth when administered before the thirtieth week of pregnancy; however, they added a pro-

---

*Nifedipine is in a class of drugs called calcium channel blockers. Nifedipine relaxes (widens) the blood vessels (veins and arteries), which makes it easier for the heart to pump and reduces its workload.

viso stating that their data came from an inadequate number of patients and therefore might not be completely accurate. This medication cannot be taken if you have stomach ulcers or if you are allergic to aspirin or ibuprofen. Physicians also limit its usage to before the thirty-second week of pregnancy, as it can negatively affect fetal circulation after this point, which can be a very serious side effect and extremely detrimental to the fetus.

• **Terbutaline.** This drug, in the class of beta-mimetics, is probably the most frequently used medication for outpatient visits. Women who are treated for preterm contractions with terbutaline often feel like they can go home and clean the entire house. This medication is structurally similar to adrenaline and thus may cause side effects like tachycardia (increased heart rate), chest discomfort, palpitations, headache, nasal congestion, and nausea and vomiting. Because of these side effects, patients usually refuse terbutaline if they have received it in the past. The Cochrane Collaboration has found that administration of this medication resulted in a decrease in patients who delivered within the first forty-eight hours. Because of the metabolic side effects of this medication, it is rarely prescribed for long-term usage. Terbutaline has been shown to increase blood sugar levels and can reduce the amount of potassium in the blood. If you are on these medications long term, your physician may order blood levels for glucose and potassium intermittently to monitor your health.

> Grace was in her thirtieth week of her fourth pregnancy when she started having uterine contractions one evening while watching television. Per our instructions, she tried increasing her amount of fluid intake and continued lying down. The contractions, however, became more regular and increased to ten-minute intervals. The pain also increased. She ended up going to the hospital, where the nurses picked up the uterine contractions on the monitor but found her cervix still closed and thick. The contractions were not strong enough to dilate her cervix. Terbutaline was ordered, and after three doses of the medication she became restless and her heart rate increased to around 100 beats per minute. Her contractions now occurred every fifteen minutes. The conundrum with terbutaline is that sometimes it will eliminate preterm contrac-

tions and other times it doesn't change a thing. If the cervix had been dilating, Grace would have been admitted to the hospital, but because the cervix remained closed, she technically wasn't in preterm labor. Grace was eventually admitted to the hospital and started on intravenous magnesium because of the pain of her contractions. After two days her medications were decreased and her contractions disappeared. She was discharged from the hospital and the remainder of her pregnancy was uneventful. As a matter of fact, she went past her due date, and we induced labor. As this story illustrates, preterm contractions do not always result in preterm birth.

Perhaps you know a woman who is going to the hospital with uterine contractions every five or six weeks. It can happen. For a while, she was accepting medications, then she started refusing them because they "don't do anything but make me feel horrible." To a certain extent she is right: no medication has been proven to extend the length of a pregnancy much beyond seven days, but medications can extend the pregnancy long enough to increase the baby's chance of survival. This is the healthcare provider's goal. We have treatments at our disposal and we will use them as necessary for those of you in preterm labor. Obstetrics is truly the only profession where there are two patients, and in the case of preterm labor we are treating you in order to help our other patient, the baby.

2. If I'm overweight, I have a decreased chance of delivering a preterm baby.

According to a study published in January 2009 in *Obstetrics & Gynecology*, overweight women have a lower incidence of preterm birth than underweight or average-sized women.[3] Overweight women had an 8 percent risk of preterm birth, while average or underweight women had a risk of almost 22 percent at each gestational age interval studied. The study defined overweight women as those with a BMI of 25 kg/m. This means that if a five-foot-five-inch-tall woman weighs more than 150 pounds, she's overweight. Ouch! First of all, let's get over the fact that this study claims you are overweight if you are 150 pounds at five foot five. Second, just because the statement above is not a myth doesn't give anyone license to eat mindlessly. Women who are overweight during pregnancy have higher rates of diabetes and high blood pressure. The added weight also stresses bones, which causes the osteoclasts to deposit more bone to help carry the weight. Thus, overweight women have lower incidences of osteoporosis. Fat is also the main component of breast milk. Overweight women may not make substantially more breast milk, but underweight women may have a problem producing adequate milk. To date, our largest patient was over 400 pounds, and she did not go into preterm labor. So while this claim is obviously not an absolute, it doesn't mean it's not better to start smaller. Fat *is* good for a few things in life. With this study, it seems that a little bit of fat can protect against preterm birth.

3. Clean and healthy teeth mean lower chances of preterm birth.

You have many reasons to smile when you're pregnant. Add another item to the list if you have healthy teeth and receive proper dental care before and during your pregnancy, because healthy teeth and gums will indeed reduce the risks of preterm birth. Aetna and Columbia University College of Dental Medicine reviewed the charts of their patients between January 2003 and September 2006. They compared 1,491 patients who received dental treatment during pregnancy with 1,172 women who did not receive any dental care during pregnancy. Dental care was considered to be either a gum treatment or regular teeth cleaning. The preterm birthrate for those women receiving dental care was 6.4 percent, while the preterm birthrate for those women not receiving dental care was 11 percent. They concluded that routine dental care benefits the health of the unborn infant. Since preterm births cost this country millions of dollars per year, Aetna found that by encouraging their members to have routine dental care before and during pregnancy, they were making an impact on the rates of preterm birth.

For every study that points one way, there is another study that negates the first study. So, in January 2009, a study of 1,800 pregnant women with periodontal disease (gum disease) assigned half of the patients to treatment, while the other half received none. The data showed no difference in preterm rates between the two groups.

Regardless of whether the data point to dental hygiene as a potential cause for preterm labor, it's a good and safe practice to have your teeth cleaned twice a year as recommended by the American Dental Association.

4. I currently have depression and I was told that depression doubles my risk of preterm labor.

Scientific research indicates that increased anxiety and depression may play a role in preterm labor. The research to date, however, remains inconclusive, making the above statement a myth. If you have untreated anxiety or depression, please consider going to a mental health professional. By doing so, you might be able to decrease risks to your physical health, and this could greatly help your baby. If you are on anxiety or depression medications and feel better when you are taking them, then we usually recommend that you stay on them with the help of your physician.

5. I need to quit my job and be on bed rest because it will decrease my chance of preterm birth.

Assuming that you have discussed this with your doctor and you are certain that your problems are not caused by something treatable like a bladder or vaginal infection, then let's send you home with a monitor and put you on bed rest. The National Institutes of Health did this very study in 2002. The study was conducted with participation from eleven large medical centers in the United States. Researchers discovered that women who were being monitored at home for contractions had no real change in the treatment of preterm labor. If a woman was having issues with preterm contractions and was sent home by her employer, the study found no increase in the likelihood of her going into labor. The home monitoring was also not able to find a specific number of contractions that increased a woman's risk. It was detected that women with more contractions overall have a higher rate of premature birth, but there was no discernable pattern to these contractions in the study. Simply putting you on bed rest will not keep you from going into preterm labor. It makes sense to think that if you slow down and take it easy, you relax and so should your uterus, but there just aren't any data to back this up. You're pregnant, not broken. You can do the work you used to do and you can even push yourself a little. While bed rest may not be the cure for preterm labor, it can help rest your joints and keep you in the game.

> When I was stationed at Reynolds Army Community Hospital in Lawton, Oklahoma, I had a pregnant patient who worked as a nurse in the ICU. She handled her twelve-hour shifts wonderfully until she hit about thirty-three weeks and then everything came to a screeching halt. Her feet and knees felt constantly sore, and she had a severe pressure in her pelvis. She weighed only one hundred and thirty pounds at the start of her pregnancy and had gained twenty-eight pounds up to this point. The increased weight was wreaking havoc on her tiny frame. I spoke with her CO (commanding officer) and asked if she could be cut down to eight-hour shifts, which I felt would be easier on her and still allow her forty hours of work a week. Her CO's response was an emphatic "No, sir." When I asked why, I was told that my patient was a soldier and this was part of her duty. I then went to the hospital commander, who granted the request.
>
> It seems my patient's CO had never been pregnant and did not truly understand the problem that an additional twenty-eight pounds of weight (in a relatively small period of time) could cause during a demanding twelve-hour shift in the ICU. I challenged the CO to wear a thirty-pound backpack during her eight-hour shift and keep it on for another four hours. She accepted the challenge. Ten days later she came to me and said, "I don't ever want to be pregnant, sir." We had a good laugh, and her conversion was such that she protected her pregnant nurse from that point on.

6. There is a cotton swab test that I can do to tell if I am likely to go into preterm labor.

Yes, there is a cotton swab test that signifies if you have an increased risk for preterm labor and birth, but it cannot be done at home. The test is called a fetal fibronectin (fFN) and it is recommended by the American College of Obstetricians and Gynecologists for women with symptoms of preterm labor. The test requires a simple cotton swab of the cervix, which must be done before a nurse or physician checks your cervix with gel. The test is invalid if you've recently had intercourse. This swab of the cervico-vaginal mucus is analyzed for fFN, a protein secreted during pregnancy that acts like an adhesive attaching the bag of water to the uterine lining. This protein is detectable up to twenty-two weeks of pregnancy and then disappears until about three weeks before your due date. The test can be done between twenty-four and thirty-four weeks. As stated earlier, the presence of fFN in the secretions means there is an increased risk of preterm delivery (61 percent before thirty-one weeks). If you test positive for fFN, this could signal that the adhesive in your uterus is breaking down. When the test comes back negative, it signifies a 95 percent chance that you will not deliver early.[4]

This test sounds worthwhile, right? So why isn't it used regularly throughout every woman's pregnancy? That's a good question, and one that has been researched. Studies have shown that routine testing of women throughout their pregnancies has not been shown to be clinically effective in reducing the rates of preterm birth. Even this test has its limitations, but it will provide good information in certain circumstances. The final item that makes this an important test is that the fFN can predict potential preterm labor even before dilation of the cervix.[5]

7. Sex can cause preterm birth.

Men frequently become concerned that sex and sexual positions can influence preterm birth, or that they might be injuring the baby during intercourse. With regard to preterm birth, there is a small chance that sex can start contractions because of two factors: the male semen and the female orgasm. The male semen contains a chemical compound called prostaglandin, a chemical used in medicinal form to induce labor. One study showed that male semen contains a wide range of amounts of prostaglandin in the semen, ranging from 2 to 272 micrograms. The amount not only varies among men but varies between one man's different ejaculations as well. The usual dose for labor induction is 25 to 50 micrograms administered vaginally as a small tablet.

The bottom-line question here is: Should you avoid intercourse if you've already had a previous pregnancy with a preterm birth? Most clinicians will advise you not to have sex if you're having preterm contractions and preterm labor. Well, what about if you've had a preterm birth in the past? In one study, 187 pregnant women between sixteen and eighteen weeks pregnant who had previously had a preterm birth were asked about their sexual history. Thirty-eight percent of the women reporting higher frequency of sex had preterm labor while 28 percent of those reporting little or no sex had preterm labor. The physicians involved in this study have stated that sexual intercourse during pregnancy is "probably okay" for women with a history of preterm birth. Listed exceptions to this rule would be those women with a cervical *cerclage* (a stitch placed in the cervix to keep it closed), ruptured membranes, or a prematurely dilated cervix. If you have a risk factor for preterm labor, it would be wise to ask your healthcare provider his or her opinion as to whether or not intercourse is safe.

> Yvonne and her husband came to the office for a routine visit with no complications, but they had a question. Yvonne looked at me and asked me to tell her husband that he wasn't hurting the baby when they had sex. Her husband looked like the Incredible Hulk, a big muscular guy that stood six foot two inches tall and weighed about two hundred and fifty pounds. After I wiped an anxious bead of sweat from my brow, I explained to him the anatomy and length of the vagina and how it can accommodate most male anatomy, and that the baby was safely hidden behind the cervix so there was no chance of him hitting the baby with his penis.
>
> "I not worried about hitting the baby with my penis, Doc," he laughed. "I'm worried that when I lie on her I'm crushing the kid."
>
> We both laughed as only a couple of men could do, and then I explained to him how the baby was safe in its bag of amniotic fluid and unless he was putting all of his weigh on her for an extended period of time, the baby wasn't feeling any of the pressure.

8. Once a preterm delivery, always a preterm delivery.

If you have experienced a preterm birth, then you know the emotional challenge of leaving the hospital without your baby, followed by the challenge of daily return trips to the hospital to provide breast milk for feedings. The bonding experience is less than ideal in these circumstances. Moreover, the sterility of the hospital is far different than the comfort of a home nursery. So what's your first worry when you become pregnant again? That you'll have to endure the entire process again, which your friend said might be the case since one preterm birth means that you'll have another.

Approximately 10 to 15 percent of women with a previous preterm birth will deliver early again. There is not much you can do about this unless there was a particular reason for the preterm labor in your previous pregnancy. For instance, some women experienced preterm labor because of lack of proper prenatal care during their last pregnancy; obviously this could be changed the second time around. Other reasons for previous preterm births are usage of alcohol or drugs, domestic violence, lack of emotional or physical support, and stress, and these are all things that you can control. In cases where there is a structural anomaly of the cervix or uterus or unknown infection, there may be nothing to be done to prevent another preterm birth.

As you can see, once a preterm birth is not always a preterm birth. Actually, the odds are in your favor that you will not have a preterm birth this time around. Make sure you get frequent and early care for your pregnancy if you have a history of preterm birth and be aware of the signs and symptoms of preterm labor. If you experience symptoms of low back pain, tightening of the stomach on a regular basis, deep pressure in the vagina, leakage of clear fluid, or vaginal bleeding, call your provider immediately. Many women who experience signs of preterm labor will go on to deliver a healthy full-term infant. No one knows your body better than you. Always let your provider know how you are doing.

9. A common vaginal infection can cause preterm labor.

This one is not myth, it's the truth. A number of vaginal infections can instigate preterm labor and contractions. The Centers for Disease Control and Prevention keep watch of this yearly with their STDs and Pregnancy Report.[6] The most recent reports show that an infection called *bacterial vaginosis* is the most common infection in pregnant women.

STDs	Estimated number of pregnant women
Bacterial vaginosis	1,080,000
Herpes simplex virus 2	880,000
Chlamydia	100,000
Trichomoniasis	140,000
Gonorrhea	13,200
Hepatitis B	16,000
HIV	6,400
Syphilis	<1,000

Statistics show that women with bacterial vaginosis infections have a higher incidence of preterm labor. A large multicenter study evaluated over 20,000 pregnant women who were screened for two types of vaginal infections: bacterial vaginosis and trichomoniasis.[7] The purpose of this study was to see if routine screening for these infections would reduce the rate of preterm labor. Of the women screened, 6,540 tested positive for bacterial vaginosis. These women were then randomized into two groups. One received the antibiotic metronidazole, while the other group received a placebo. Researchers determined that the women treated with metronidazole did not experience fewer hospital admissions for preterm labor, neonatal admissions to ICU, receipt of preterm labor medications, or neonatal death, despite proof that metronidazole effectively treats bacterial vaginosis (cure rate of approximately 78 percent in this study). These results conflict with those reported in earlier studies that showed antibiotics (specifically metronidazole and erythromycin) did prevent preterm birth.

Other infections that can cause preterm labor include *asymptomatic bacteruria*, the equivalent to a bladder infection without symptoms, which occurs in 7 to 10 percent of pregnancies.[8] Chlamydia is another stealthy infection that often does not leave a trail of symptoms. Many patients come to the office for their initial OB visit and after routine testing discover they have chlamydia. Treatment is a must in order to protect your baby from preterm labor. In addition, if the baby is born through the cervix and vagina of a woman with chlamydia, there is a chance that the baby's eyes could become infected. That's why nurses automatically put antibiotics in babies' eyes at birth. Finally, gonorrhea is a sexually transmitted bacteria that can cause cervical infection and preterm labor. Gonorrhea can be detected by pap smear, or your doctor will test you at some point in the first trimester, and possibly recheck in the third trimester. If you are positive for gonorrhea, it is recommended that you receive treatment and your partner be tested and treated as well.

10. Strenuous physical activity will initiate preterm labor.

Physical activities can bring on preterm labor symptoms in some women. If any symptoms begin while you are doing any of these activities, stop doing them until you talk to your healthcare provider.

> **Sports.** Running, jogging, aerobics, bike riding, and other active sports can cause problems for some women. If you feel symptoms, stop until you talk to your provider.
>
> **Climbing stairs.** If you find that several trips up and down the stairs each day brings on preterm labor symptoms, try to organize your tasks so you make only one trip down and one trip up each day.
>
> **Heavy lifting.** Carrying groceries or laundry baskets or toting heavy toddlers can start preterm symptoms in some women. Ask someone to help you. Avoid carrying your toddler by using a stroller, asking the child to walk, or sitting rather than standing with him or her in your arms.
>
> **Heavy housework.** Scrubbing floors, washing walls, or any other strenuous housework may have to wait until after the baby is born. Lighter housework can be adjusted if you feel any symptoms. Try sitting down when you iron or fold clothes or prepare food for cooking.

Thankfully, most women will not experience preterm delivery. Preterm contractions, on the other hand, are frequent and something you should be aware of after your twentieth week of gestation. The purpose of this chapter is to alert you to common issues associated with preterm contractions, preterm labor, and possible risks of preterm birth and to distill these issues from predominant myths. Knowledge has a way of reducing fear; no one wants to spend her pregnancy entrenched in fear and worry. Plus, when you understand what is happening to your body, you can work in tandem with your physician or healthcare provider, and it is no myth that he wants to do whatever is in the best interest of you and your baby.

Notes

1. http://www.healthline.com/yodocontent/pregnancy/preterm-labor -adjunctive-therapy.html (accessed January 17, 2009).

2. R. L. Goldberg et al., "Epidemiology and Causes of Preterm Birth," *Lancet* 371(2008): 75.

3. H. M. Ehrenberg et al., "Maternal Obesity, Uterine Activity, and the Risk of Spontaneous Preterm Birth," *Obstetrics & Gynecology* 113, no. 1 (2009): 48.

4. American College of Obstetrics and Gynecology, "Assessment of Risk Factors for Preterm Birth," *Obstetrics & Gynecology* 98, no. 4 (2001): 709.

5. H. Honest et al., "Accuracy of Cervicovaginal Fetal Fibronectin Test in Predicting Risk of Spontaneous Preterm Birth: Systematic Review," *British Medical Journal* 325 (2002): 301; J. D. Iams, "Prediction and Early Detection of Preterm Labor," *Obstetrics & Gynecology* 101, no. 2 (2003): 402.

6. http://www.cdc.gov/STD/STDFact-STDs&Pregnancy.htm (accessed January 20, 2009).

7. J. Christopher Carey et al., "Metronidazole to Prevent Preterm Delivery in Pregnant Women with Asymptomatic Bacterial Vaginosis," *New England Journal of Medicine* 342 (2000): 534.

8. US Preventive Services Task Force, *Guide to Clinical Preventive Services: Report of the U.S. Preventive Services Task Force*, 2nd ed. (Baltimore: Williams & Wilkins, 1996).

Chapter Nine

Delivery Room Myths
Debunking the Delivery Room

᙭ᖇᖚ

You've made it through the nausea and vomiting of the first trimester and the smooth sailing of the second trimester. You've even weathered the trying third trimester.

What happens next?

The delivery.

In the majority of cases today, women deliver in hospitals. Some expectant mothers, however, still choose either a home birth or a delivery in a birthing center with a midwife. Many people have strong opinions on just where a woman should deliver, whether it is a physician questioning the use of doulas and home birthing, or a midwife claiming that most hospital deliveries are unnecessary. There are many different ways and places to deliver a baby. Because a majority of women choose to deliver in a hospital setting, many myths have been propagated throughout the years about a hospital birth.

The purpose of this chapter is to explain the hospital delivery room process. We are not claiming that this is the only birthing option, but it's the process that we know best and is the one in which the majority of this country's physicians participate. As physicians, we realize we may have biases ourselves, but we also understand that each woman has her own needs and desires. Above all, we feel that you, the patient, should actively seek out a physician, midwife, or doula with whom you share a strong rapport and mutual trust, as well as a facility that provides you the most comfort.

One further thought regarding the hospital birthing process. There are definitely people who feel that our current healthcare system lacks respect for the birthing process, that it's impatient and cold. Because our healthcare is rooted in a paradigm that encourages regulation and litigation, the system tends toward the defensive and impersonal. Moreover, as our country progresses toward safer births, medical procedures and treatments tend to become more invasive. Neonatologists, for instance, have the ability to save a fetus born after only twenty-four weeks of gestation, which is one example that brings us to ethical boundaries, increased costs, and suboptimal outcomes. The system has created a hospital environment that aggressively prolongs and extends life but that has also become less humane and seemingly less respectful of the natural process.

Katherine Fallon, mother and author, summoned up these sentiments in an online article:

> Within the past century, there has been tremendous importance placed on making it to the hospital. It is now being argued that it may have been better for myself and my mother if I had been born in the front seat of that tiny car. A lot of frightening statistics and personal stories about negative experiences with hospital care have recently been brought to light. The largest issue surrounding hospital deliveries is that of the frequency with which they turn to cesarean sections as an alternative to time-consuming vaginal births. In hospitals, women have a one-in-four chance of cesarean section. The lack of concern for a woman's natural birth process, along with the dangers associated with repeated cesarean sections, creates a highly volatile situation in which many women have begun to voice their objections, offering midwifery and home birth as hopeful alternatives.[1]

If you look carefully at Fallon's argument, certain phrases stand out: "negative experiences," "time-consuming vaginal births," "lack of concern," "highly volatile." These words confer the author's apparent distrust for the current medical system. The problem is that not all physicians and medical facilities fit into this negatively constructed box. It's true that approximately 25 percent of deliveries today are by cesarean section. Yet if you exclude those women who choose to have a cesarean section because they had one in the past, this rate decreases to approximately 10 to 12 percent. As always, language and statistics run the risk of reflecting bias, depending on the way they are presented. While we disagree with Fallon's insights, we can also appreciate how the healthcare system seems to foster some of these negative feelings. The purpose of this chapter is to explore some common delivery room myths and statistics and in so doing, shed light and understanding on them.

1. When I arrive at the hospital, I will be greeted with a shave and an enema.

In the last fifteen years, neither of us has witnessed a patient being shaved or given an enema. It would be within your right as a patient to request either of these procedures, but it certainly isn't standard practice. Still, patients continue to ask us if they will be shaved at the hospital or if they will need to shave themselves before coming to the hospital. Shaving pubic hair is not necessary; in fact, doing so can increase infection rates if done with a razor and not surgical clippers. Occasionally, the pubic hair may be trimmed with clippers in the operating room prior to a cesarean section, but only at the discretion of the surgeon, and usually only if the hair will cover the incision. Multiple studies have actually confirmed that shaving with a razor over or around surgical sites may increase the risk of infection.[2] This is not to say that you can't or shouldn't shave prior to your delivery. It just isn't necessary. These days, we find that many women perform laser hair removal or wax or shave their pubic area even when they aren't pregnant, so this is less of a concern than it used to be.

Patients also ask if they will need to undergo an enema when they are brought to the hospital in labor. In the past, it was thought that enemas were necessary to evacuate the rectum and the lower colon of feces in order to decrease infection rates. Studies have shown that there is no difference in rates of perineal infection in the mother or of upper respiratory infections to the infant. Furthermore, there was no difference in patient satisfaction with their delivery experience, either with or without an enema.[3] So the answer is no, you do not need to undergo an enema before or during labor.

2. I need to have a birth plan prior to arriving at the hospital, or I will be at the mercy of the physician and hospital policy.

Let's keep in mind the fact that every labor is unique. Physicians may follow certain protocols for inducing labor augmentation (assisting the progress of labor with medication) or performing a cesarean section. These protocols take into consideration the need for specific items and procedures such as intravenous fluids, blood tests, fetal monitoring, pain medications, and antibiotics. Protocols, however, are not written in indelible ink. They can and should be changed based on each individual patient's needs.

We suggest that you discuss the following topics with your physician or midwife prior to coming to the hospital. Just as every woman is different, every provider is different. Therefore, it's important for you to understand your provider's philosophy regarding labor and delivery. There are definitely variations.

- Who is your labor coach?
- How will you set up the delivery room: Will you use music or aromatherapy? Who will be there and for which parts of your labor and delivery?
- Do you want the ability to be mobile while you are in labor?
- What is your plan for pain management? (i.e., Lamaze, IV narcotics, epidural)
- Do you or a family member wish to cut the cord?
- Will you want the baby to go directly to your belly after the birth?
- Are you going to breastfeed or will you bottle-feed the baby?

You may have other wishes or needs to add to this list. If you do, make sure you address all items that are important to you prior to labor. Everyone wants to avoid surprises in the delivery room.

K. B. was a thirty-nine-year-old litigation attorney married to an engineer who came to see me at five weeks of pregnancy, her first pregnancy. As I recall, that first visit, the one in which we get acquainted and take a complete history and do a full physical exam, she wanted to discuss her birthing plan. She was a planner, and she knew it, and she wanted me to know it too. She let me know that day that she was planning on using the Bradley method, a partner-coached labor and delivery method that emphasizes natural childbirth. By thirty-nine weeks I knew K. B. very well and I was well informed about every possible detail of her upcoming delivery. She was an attractive, highly intelligent, and very pleasant individual with a very supportive and loving husband. He came to each and every appointment, and their excitement was palpable at each visit. I looked forward to their delivery.

One night she came to labor and delivery because her bag of water had broken. This is an indication that you come to the hospital, not so much because labor is imminent, but because the barrier between the baby and the outside world has been broken and the baby is now at risk for infection. K. B. came in with her doula and her music and her aromatherapy—and her husband, of course. She was well equipped for her desired natural birth. She began having contractions right away, actually, but unfortunately, her cervix was only dilated to 1 cm. After twenty-four hours her cervix had dilated to only 4 cm, which can happen with a first-time mother. She was a little disheartened, in a great deal of pain, and starting to get tired, but she was determined to persevere. Her support remained encouraging for her as always. At this point, her labor stalled significantly, and, despite that, she was still in a great deal of pain. Her contractions were very strong but not dilating her cervix. She was almost inconsolable at this point but very determined not to take any medication for the pain and definitely did not want an epidural. But at this point the music and the pleasant smells of the aromatherapy, and the gentle massages from her husband were not even touching her complete and utter exhaustion. It had been thirty-six hours of intense pain. The room was starting to look dirty. The sheets disheveled, empty cups everywhere, . . . no more music. Things were definitely not turning out the way she had been planning over the last nine months.

Then the baby started showing signs of infection, and K. B. began to run a temperature. She was yelling at her husband and then asked for the epidural. She was still dilating, although very slowly. At this point, she was only 6 cm, and it could be hours until she could start pushing—too long to wait given the fever and the baby's signs of infection. We gave her antibiotics and Tylenol to bring the fever down, but the signs of infection were worsening. I recommended a C-section. Through her tears of exhaustion and her sheer disappointment, she agreed, as she wanted what was safest for the baby. The C-section went very well, and she delivered a beautiful baby girl. After her surgery, she had a sense of serene calm about her, in direct contrast to the hour before. She was overjoyed by her new baby and so grateful for all the help she received. No, it wasn't the way she planned, but she smiled up at me and with tears of gratitude said, "I should have known, shouldn't I?"

I share this with you not to scare you but to highlight the point that childbirth does not always follow our careful plans. Many aspects of delivery are out of your control, and no amount of planning is going to change that. So the lesson here is to be prepared for anything. Just as in life, so in birth.

3. My doctor has admitted me to labor and delivery for induction of labor. I'm afraid, because I've heard that being induced hurts more than natural labor.

Labor is a painful process. One or two women out there might argue this, but we think it's safe to say that labor is painful across the board. As far as induction, we would hope that you are not being induced without your consent. No medical procedure, including an induction of labor, can take place without a patient's consent.

There are multiple reasons for inducing labor. Sometimes the patient requests induction. A family member may be coming from out of town, or the patient may be suffering extreme discomfort. Physicians may recommend that a patient be induced for medical reasons, such as preeclampsia (rise in blood pressure, protein in the urine, and edema), decreased amniotic fluid (oligohydramnios), intrauterine growth restriction,* twins, and gestational diabetes.

Just as there are multiple indications for labor induction, there are also multiple means by which to induce. Your physician or provider will determine which method is best by using a system called the Bishop's score. This score helps predict how likely your cervix is to dilate with an induction. The word *ripe* is used to indicate that the cervix is ready to dilate. In

---

*Intrauterine growth restriction, or IUGR, is the term used when an infant is below the 10th percentile for weight at its given gestational age. This is usually calculated by ultrasound, and while there can be errors in ultrasonographic measurements, physicians will usually see a trend in the fetal growth. For instance, your baby may be in the 43rd percentile at 28 weeks, the 32nd percentile at 32 weeks, the 15th percentile at 35 weeks, and the 5th percentile at 38 weeks. This pattern shows a definite restriction in the growth process.

other words, it will be more receptive to dilation when induced. The scoring system takes into account the following factors:

- **Cervical dilation.** The opening of the cervix is measured in centimeters, ranging from 0 (closed) to 10.
- **Cervical effacement.** This term describes the thinning and shortening of the cervix. A cervix less receptive to induction is long and thick, whereas a ripened cervix is thinner. Cervical effacement is described in terms of percentage. A normal, long cervix is approximately 4 centimeters in length. If it is 50 percent effaced, it's approximately 2 centimeters in length; 100 percent effacement means the cervix is as thin as paper.
- **Station of the fetal head.** The station measures the location of the tip of the fetal skull in relation to the bony prominences of the maternal pelvis called the *ischial spines*. Zero station occurs when the fetal head is at the level of the spines. When the fetal head is crowning and visible at the perineum, the station is +5 station. A −5 station, on the other hand, means that the fetal head is floating in amniotic fluid and is not engaged in the pelvis. This fetal position is called *ballotable*. So, the lower the station, the more ripe the cervix.
- **Position of the cervix in the vagina.** When the cervix points toward the back of the vagina, it's in a posterior position. When it points to the front of the vagina, it's called anterior, and when it points to the opening of the vagina, it's midline. Midline and anterior cervixes are considered ripe. The cervix will move more toward the vaginal opening when it is ready for labor.
- **Cervical consistency.** Normally a cervix feels like the tip of your nose. If the cervix is soft, like the texture of your cheek, it is considered ripened and ready for induction.

Each portion of the Bishop's score can receive a 0, 1, 2, or 3. A cumulative score of 8 or more is likely to support a successful induction.[4] If the Bishop's score is low, indicating that the cervix is not as susceptible to dilation, a medication will be used to ripen it. Vaginal pills or gels may be used, as well as medications on a string that can be inserted into the vagina. Typically, these methods do not initiate painful contractions and are well tolerated. Once the cervix changes in dilation, position, or consistency, Pitocin (brand name of oxytocin) will be administered. In many cases, if the cervix is already considered ripe, induction will start immediately with intravenous oxytocin. Sometimes, breaking the bag of water, which is technically called artificial rupture of membranes, is used in combination with Pitocin. Occasionally a labor becomes dysfunctional, meaning that contractions are irregular and the cervix is not dilating. In this case, labor is "augmented" with Pitocin in order to obtain "functional labor," meaning that contractions will cause the cervix to dilate and ultimately result in the safe delivery of the infant.

Many women think that contractions induced by Pitocin are more painful than those of regular labor. This must be the gist of why so many women think that an induction hurts more than going into labor naturally. Is this merely a misguided perception or do contractions brought on by Pitocin really hurt more than natural contractions? The Pitocin used intravenously during labor and delivery is biologically identical to the Pitocin—called oxytocin—made by your pituitary gland. Contractions stimulated through intravenous Pitocin may possibly affect the uterus in a different manner than natural labor, though this has not been proven.

If a patient experiences dysfunctional labor, as described above, we may augment her labor with Pitocin, which will result in a functional labor. As the labor begins to progress normally, the pain also begins. The Pitocin itself does not cause pain; it increases the frequency and power of contractions, thereby increasing discomfort.

Another reason for the perception that induction results in more pain has to do with the stages of labor. Labor includes two phases: a latent phase and an active phase. The latent phase occurs at the very beginning of labor and can last anywhere from twenty-four to forty-eight hours for a first pregnancy. It is signaled by contractions that are irregular but persistent and a cervix that is dilated anywhere from 1 to 4 centimeters. The active phase of labor starts when the cervix is dilated to at least 4 centimeters and regular contractions occur at least every five minutes.

Usually women who go into labor naturally are told to come to the hospital when their contractions are five minutes apart and they have difficulty talking during them. When contractions occur at this interval, the patient is likely to be in active labor. When a patient is induced, she may be "stuck" in the latent phase, which means being in the hospital for a longer period of time while the medication is beginning to work on the uterus and cervix. If not induced, a patient is at home during this period, in the comfort of her own bed and able to move around and eat or drink. Conversely, the induced patient is in the hospital, typically in bed and hooked up to a fetal monitor. Perhaps this difference is one reason why induction is perceived as being more painful.

Furthermore, once labor becomes active and functional, meaning the cervix is dilating and the contractions are consistent, it becomes painful. So whether active labor occurs by the natural secretion of your own Pitocin, or the injection of Pitocin intravenously, as in an induction, it hurts.

All of these factors likely contribute to the perception that induction "hurts" more than spontaneous labor. As a male obstetrician, Shawn can honestly say that he has never experienced labor, but we have both witnessed labor in thousands of cases, and be it natural or induced, it hurts.

4. The labor and delivery ward will be especially busy around my due date because it's during a full moon.

Myths surrounding the full moon and the weird behaviors blamed upon it prevail worldwide. The full moon has been linked to everything from increased criminal behavior to increased birthrates. We often hear nurses stating that tomorrow will be busy because of the full moon. One study actually evaluated individual behaviors and their relationship to the lunar cycle. The researchers discovered that, contrary to popular belief, the phases of the moon did not increase the following incidents:

- Homicidal rate
- Traffic accidents
- Crisis calls to police or fire stations
- Domestic violence
- Births of babies
- Suicide rates
- Major disasters
- Casino payout rates
- Assassinations
- Kidnappings
- Aggression by professional hockey players
- Violence in prisons

- Psychiatric admissions
- Agitated behavior by nursing home residents
- Gunshot wounds
- Stabbings
- Emergency room admissions
- Alcoholic behavior
- Sleepwalking[5]

In addition, a study analyzed the birthdays of 4,256 babies born in a clinic in France and found the deliveries equally distributed throughout the phases of the lunar cycle.[6] Another study done in Italy evaluated 7,842 spontaneous deliveries and found no relationship between the number of babies born and lunar cycles.

The moon may pull on the ocean tides and affect the habits or moods of some individuals, but it does not appear to influence the delivery rates at hospitals.

5. Epidurals can cause nerve damage or paralysis.

During the course of labor, many women choose to have some sort of pain control. Of those women, a majority will opt for epidural anesthesia.

> While practicing obstetrics in the military system, I was assigned the task of teaching a birthing class at the hospital. During the first discussion of epidural anesthesia, I decided to conduct an informal study on the patients and their desires for anesthesia, if any. I placed ten sheets of paper numbered one through ten in sequential order on the floor. I then asked the patients to stand behind a certain number. Patients completely opposed to epidural anesthesia stood behind number one and those definite about using an epidural stood behind number ten. Patients uncertain about epidurals stood behind a number in between. As I repeated this exercise with each class, I discovered consistent desires on the part of patients. Eighty to 90 percent would line up behind number one, while 10 to 20 percent of patients would stand behind number ten. What fascinated me was that nobody ever stood behind the numbers in between. This simple study shows how polarizing this issue can be and how intensely ingrained we are in our individual belief structures.

There are hundreds of reasons for having a natural childbirth. If you have a strong desire to experience this, we would certainly encourage it. If the reason for a natural birth, meaning one without pain medication or epidural, is a fear of the epidural itself, then please read ahead with an open mind. Many women fear that the epidural will cause nerve damage or paralysis. This fear usually stems from a story related by a friend or family member.

The first recorded use of an epidural was in 1885 in New York when neurologist J. Leonard Corning injected cocaine into the epidural space of a patient suffering from "spinal weakness seminal incontinence."[7] Recent studies from 2002 show that approximately 66 percent of women used epidural anesthesia, and more than half of those patients had vaginal deliveries.[8] Interestingly, utilization of epidurals has not increased patient satisfaction with the birthing process.[9] Epidurals can influence and affect the birthing hormones by decreasing the pain sensation, but studies have shown that epidurals decrease levels of naturally produced beta-endorphins, which are the body's natural narcotics.

What are the side effects of epidurals, and can they harm or paralyze you? Keep in mind that any surgical procedure—and we consider the placement of an epidural a minor surgical procedure, carries risks and benefits. We would like to remind the reader that these risks are rare. Since epidurals are elective procedures, you should have an extensive consent process, meaning that you should speak with the practitioner who will be inserting the epidural catheter and ask all your questions of him or her.

The following is a list of epidural complications, presented in no particular order:

- Hypotension, or a significant drop in the patient's blood pressure, can be seen in almost half of the epidurals placed.[10]
- Sedation occurs in 20 percent of women.[11]
- Nausea and vomiting occur in 1 out of 20 patients.
- Inadequate pain control happens in 10 to 15 percent of patients. This number reflects the patient who has a desire for 100 percent pain control, which, under perfect conditions, may be impossible to obtain. Remember, epidurals are an elective procedure for pain control, not necessarily pain elimination.
- Spinal headache. Approximately 1 percent of patient's receiving an epidural will incur a spinal headache. This complication results from

the tip of the needle puncturing the inner lining of the sheath covering the spinal cord. Cerebrospinal fluid can leak out, causing a headache. Patients with spinal headaches have severe migrainelike head pain when they sit upright or stand. The pain tends to improve significantly when the patient lies down. Initial treatments are aggressive hydration by mouth and increased caffeine intake. If the symptoms are severe or persistent, the physician may prescribe a blood patch. The anesthesiologist will draw a small amount of the patient's blood from the arm and inject it into the epidural site. This blood bathes the puncture site and clots over it, thus closing the hole that is leaking. Relief is usually immediate.

- Weakness and numbness after the procedure.[12] If this rare complication occurs, it's usually noticed after delivery. The actual occurrence is anywhere from 4 to 18 per 10,000 patients. In most cases the condition completely resolves within three months of the procedure. The complication results when the needle comes in contact with either the spinal cord or the nerves that enter the spinal cord. At the point where the epidural is placed, the spinal cord is not the thick cord that it is higher up in the back. It's called the *cauda equine*, Latin for "horse's tail." As the name indicates, this part of the spinal cord is a fanned-out group of very small cords, like the hair of a horse's tail. This formation increases the likelihood of injury compared to what it would be higher up where the cord is much thicker.

- Permanent disability. A retrospective study of serious nonfatal complications of epidural block in obstetric practice was carried out using a postal questionnaire. Two hundred and thirty-three obstetric units in the United Kingdom (responsible for 2,580,000 deliveries from 1982 to 1986) responded. Out of 505,000 epidural blocks performed (84 percent for pain relief and 15 percent for cesarean section), 108, or 0.0002 percent of cases involved complications, and of these 108, only 5 resulted in permanent disability. Indeed, this is an extremely rare event, a 0.000001 percent chance, to be exact.

Many women are concerned that an epidural is the only choice for pain relief during labor, which often exacerbates their fear and anxiety about labor. As discussed above, epidurals are safe, but they are not without complications. Other options for laboring patients include IV pain medications like morphine, Demerol, Stadol, and Nubain. These medications are all considered to be narcotic sedatives and cross the placenta into the fetus. Women who receive these medications claim that they can still feel pain but that they aren't overwhelmed by it and thus may be more relaxed and less fearful. Also, these medications can make the mother lightheaded and sleepy. These same symptoms can occur in the fetus and are evident with the fetal heart rate tracing. The symptoms are temporary in the mother, and the fetus's symptoms will spontaneously resolve with time. As the labor nears delivery, we stop administering these medications because they can cause respiratory depression in the newborn. This means that during the last portion of labor, as well as during the second stage of labor, which is the pushing stage, these medications are not an option for pain control.

Hypnosis has become more and more popular as a method of pain control in American hospitals. Like the Lamaze Method, hypnosis uses a focused state of concentration. Other nonmedical, natural methods of dealing with pain include the Bradley method, which teaches the mother and her partner the physiology behind labor and how to work as a team, with the partner as coach. Some women rely on a doula during labor. Literally translated from ancient Greek, *doula* means "woman who serves." Doulas provide emotional and physical support to a patient during labor and the postpartum period. We know women who used massage therapy as well as aromatherapy. We have not personally seen acupuncture used in the delivery room, and that may be because the use of needles in the delivery room would be against hospital policy. We are firm believers in complementary practices such as acupuncture, however, and hope that in the future, this practice will make its way into routine deliveries.

6. I don't want to deliver on a Friday because my baby will have depression.

Remember the nursery rhyme that assigns children attributes based on the weekday on which they were born? The original poem goes like this:

> Monday's child is fair of face.
> Tuesday's child is full of grace.
> Wednesday's child is loving and giving.

Thursday's child works hard for a living.
Friday's child is full of woe.
Saturday's child has far to go.
But the child that is born on Sabbath-day
Is bonny and happy and wise and gay.

The poem is credited to Thomas Nashe (1567–1601), a satirist and poet. It embodies the superstition that one's luck or personality is linked to a day of the week.

This nursery rhyme may be rooted in the Gregorian calendar that we use today. In the Judeo-Christian tradition, Mondays are the second day of the week, the day when saints are recognized. If there is a connection to the historical recognition of angels, then it would be natural to see how Monday's child came to be fair of face. Fridays are considered an unlucky day in Christian culture, particularly because the death of Christ occurred on a Friday. A maritime superstition attests to the bad luck of sailing on a Friday. In our modern times, superstition still surrounds Friday the thirteenth. Perhaps these views about Friday propagate the myth of Friday's child being full of woe.

Biologically and scientifically, no relationship exists between the day of the week and the personality of the infant. Certainly, ancient astrological beliefs might refute that statement, but those are more specific to time and place than simply the day of the week.

7. If I follow the Lamaze Method, I will have a pain-free delivery.

According to the Lamaze International Web site, this form of birthing process was started in 1951 by Dr. Fernand Lamaze after he witnessed it being done in Russia. The primary concepts of the Lamaze Method center around relaxation, patient education, breathing techniques, and emotional support provided by a birthing partner or trained nurse. During the late 1950s, the Lamaze Method spread to the United States, mainly because of the book *Thank You, Dr. Lamaze*, which described the birthing process of Marjorie Karmel and the assistance given by Dr. Lamaze. At the center of Lamaze is the Lamaze Philosophy of Birth:

- Birth is normal, natural, and healthy.
- The experience of birth profoundly affects women and their families.
- Women's inner wisdom guides them through birth.
- Women's confidence and ability to give birth is either enhanced or diminished by the care provider and place of birth.
- Women have the right to give birth free from routine medical interventions.
- Birth can take place safely in homes, birth centers, and hospitals.
- Childbirth education empowers women to make informed choices in healthcare, to assume responsibility for their health, and to trust their inner wisdom.[13]

Lamaze does not promise a painless birth but rather regards pain as providing a certain protection as the woman moves during the painful contractions. Women can expect a more controlled labor and delivery with Lamaze, which acts as a kind of biofeedback, helping women to breathe with the contractions and focus on the labor. The most recent literature on pregnancy includes a meta-analysis showing insufficient evidence that this type of person-to-person education decreases pain in labor.[14] Obviously, there are no drawbacks to taking childbirth classes, and we highly recommend them. In the end, the best predictor of how a woman is going to experience and cope with labor pain is her own level of self-confidence.

You won't know what to expect until you get into the active stage of labor, but you can try to familiarize yourself with the process. We would also recommend that you familiarize yourself with the hospital and your physician's protocols for calling after hours so that there are no surprises.

8. I have heard that labor is easier if I lie on my back.

According to the *American Journal of Family Practice*, the most common position for a hospital labor is lithotomy: the woman lies on her back with her legs in stirrups, knees and hips flexed. There are other acceptable, possibly even better positions in which to give birth.

Because labor typically lasts much longer than the pushing stage, a woman has ample time to walk around or get into any position that is comfortable for her as long as the bag of water remains intact and the fetus is not compromised.

Some women prefer to lie on their side with a pillow in between their legs, as this seems to help take pressure off the lower back and buttocks.

Sitting with one foot up on a chair or a sofa with the other foot on the floor will help stretch the lower back and open the pelvis. This position may be particularly helpful for women who experience contraction pains more on one side than the other, as it will allow the musculature to stretch.

In the early stages of labor, some women may find it more comfortable to stand or sway back and forth. Sitting in a rocking chair or on a birthing ball during the early stages of labor can relieve pressure from the lower back and allow the woman to concentrate on a focal point. A focal point can be anything from a picture on the wall, a piece of furniture, or her toes. Rocking or swaying has a rhythmic effect that can be useful as a means of initiating a breathing pattern.

Occasionally women feel more comfortable when they can walk around the delivery room or hallway. For some, confinement to the bed restricts the natural movement of the body and may cause feelings of anxiety. The freedom to walk logically aids the gravitational force so as to push the baby's head into the pelvis naturally. As physicians, we prefer that the patient not walk after the bag of water (chorion) has been broken, because the umbilical cord could slip past the baby's head and fall into the vagina. When this happens, the baby's blood supply and oxygen are cut off.

As mentioned, the standard position for delivering a baby in the hospital is the lithotomy position, where the woman is on her back with head slightly elevated and legs flexed against the belly. Pulling the legs toward the belly is called the McRobert's maneuver and opens the pelvic outlet to allow the fetal head and shoulders more space.

Ultimately, in situations where fetal well-being is established and the baby is considered stable and happy, whatever position of labor that is most comfortable would be ideal. As we have discussed earlier, the left lateral recumbent position (lying on the left side) maximizes blood flow to the placenta and baby. Depending on the position of the umbilical cord and whether it's wrapped around a body part in utero, other positions may be better for the fetus.

9. My uterus will do all the work.

It's long been understood that labor involves three stages. The first stage extends from the start of uterine contractions that cause significant change in the cervix to complete cervical dilation (10 centimeters). The second stage of labor begins with complete dilation of the cervix and ends with delivery of the baby, and the third stage of labor is delivery of the placenta.

The first stage of labor is completely dependent on the power of the uterus. So it's true, your uterus will do all the work, at least in this stage of labor. In most cases the uterus will exert enough power to pull and open the cervix. If this stage progresses too slowly, Pitocin may be given intra-venously to help the uterus contract more powerfully as it attempts to dilate the cervix. Physicians expect most first-time mothers, also called primi-parous patients, to dilate up to 1 centimeter per hour when they are actively in labor, while second- and third-time mothers, called multiparous patients, will dilate at a rate of 1.5 centimeters per hour. Many physicians add Pitocin for augmentation of labor if this dilation requirement isn't being met in order to stay on the path to progress and eliminate any possible com-plications with a prolonged labor. This is called active management of labor. Again, during this stage of labor, the uterus does all the work.

The second stage of labor is the time when most women begin to push. This stage can last up to three hours in primiparous women with an epidural and up to two hours in women without an epidural and in multi-parous women. Generally the epidural can add time to the second stage of labor if the woman cannot coordinate her pelvic muscles because of numbness and the absence of pain. So will your uterus do all of the work? Do you have to push? There is a concept, mainly within natural birthing circles, called "laboring down." This refers to the process of allowing the uterus to push the baby farther down into the birth canal with no effort from the mother. A number of studies have shown that continuous bearing down, or pushing, is not harmful to the fetus.[15] Other studies indicate that "laboring down," or allowing the uterus to push the baby down into the pelvis without maternal effort, is safe and should be utilized as another route of care for women in labor.[16]

Again, it may be a combination of both methods that works for one patient versus another. For women who feel a significant urge to push, having them do so not only helps them, but also may decrease their time in labor. In those women with a normal labor pattern and a stable baby, laboring down may save time and energy that would have been spent actively pushing. In addition, maternal exhaustion may be avoided by decreasing pushing time. Some medical professionals feel that laboring down decreases the amount of vaginal trauma, although this has not been proven.

10. Birth defects are caused mainly by environmental toxins.

Occasionally during the delivery process, a birth defect like cleft lip is discovered, which went undetected on antenatal ultrasound. In these instances, the parents, who are dealing with an unexpected outcome, may instinctively look for something the mother may have been exposed to during pregnancy. Without a doubt, certain environmental toxins can cause a plethora of birth defects, but many birth defects are considered multifactorial, meaning that multiple causes contributed to the process rather than one specific cause.

Birth defects, also called congenital anomalies, can range from mild to very severe and not compatible with life, meaning the baby may not live. The main causes of birth defects are environmental exposures and genetics. Many times the causes are unknown. Birth defects are seen in all parts of the world. The "background rate" for birth defects has been reported as 3 to 4 percent in the general population. This means that anyone has a 3 to 4 percent chance of having a baby with a birth defect.

Here is a short list of possible environmental or external exposures that can contribute to congenital anomalies:

- **Medications.** Accutane, Coumadin, alcohol, valproic acid
- **Infections.** German measles, toxoplasmosis, cytomegalovirus, herpes simplex
- **Maternal disease.** Diabetes
- **Heat.** Fever, external prolonged heat exposure
- **Heavy metals.** Lead, mercury

Another major cause of birth defects is chromosomal or genetic in nature and thereby hereditary. When there is suspicion of potential birth defects caused from a chromosomal or genetic transmission, there are early prenatal tests that can be performed to aid in the diagnosis. The following is a list of early prenatal testing for some congenital anomalies:

- **Alpha-fetoprotein.** This protein is secreted by the fetal liver and will be at abnormal levels in certain spinal cord and abdominal wall defects. With a Tetra Screen, the alpha-fetoprotein is drawn in addition to a human chorionic gonadotropin (hCG), estriol, and inhibin. During pregnancy, the estriol and inhibin levels are altered by the placental tissue. This level, depending on the laboratory, can be drawn from maternal blood between the fifteenth and twenty-first week.
- **Chorionic villus sampling (CVS).** Chorionic villus sampling is a sampling of the placental tissue early in the gestation. This tissue is then tested for chromosomal anomalies. This test is usually done between the tenth and thirteenth week, which is earlier than amniocentesis, discussed below. The tissue sample is obtained by inserting a needle through the maternal abdomen and then through the uterus into the placenta. It can also be performed by inserting the needle through the cervix rather than the abdomen. Because of its invasive nature, this procedure carries an increased risk of miscarriage or fetal mortality of 0.2 to 0.3 percent. CVS will not detect all congenital anomalies. On occasion some of the cells within one sample may be abnormal while others are normal. Many of these cases prove to have normal gestations. Because CVS testing is not as commonly done as amniocentesis, you should find an institution with significant experience in performing the required procedure. This testing should be reserved for those pregnancies where the earliest possible detection of an anomaly is imperative to the parents and the risks are outweighed by the benefits.
- **Amniocentesis.** This procedure involves inserting a hollow needle through the abdomen and uterus into the amniotic fluid. Approximately 5 to 10 cc of fluid is removed and sent to a lab for evaluation of fetal skin cells that are floating in the fluid. Chromosomes from these cells are evaluated for chromosomal integrity and number. Amniocentesis can be performed for chromosomal study, to evaluate for infection, to determine a spinal cord defect such as spina bifida, and to evaluate fetal lung maturity in the third trimester. The risk of

miscarriage following this procedure is approximately 1 in 200, but some feel it may actually be more like 1 in 600.[17] While this test is done later than CVS, it is generally deemed safer than CVS. Amniocentesis is performed between the twelfth and fourteenth weeks but can be performed at any time during the pregnancy with similar risks. In the latter half of the second trimester, the risks of puncturing the placenta, umbilical cord, and fetus are greater, but the procedure is still deemed safe under the proper protocols.

11. Anything that causes a birth defect in animals will do the same in humans.

As we mentioned, when unexpected birth defects are present at the time of birth, parents and families tend to blame a variety of superstitions and myths as they come to terms with the condition of their newborn baby. The mother, for instance, may try to recall whether she ingested something during her pregnancy that could be responsible for the defect. Commonly, over-the-counter medications will warn against consumption during pregnancy. Most of the time, this disclaimer exists for the legal protection of the manufacturer.

So what really constitutes a risk? The pregnancy risk category is an assessment of the potential risk that a pharmaceutical agent poses to the fetus. Pregnancy categories are usually included in the voluminous small print of the package insert. Different countries may use different criteria to define pregnancy risk categories; we will be discussing those categories set by the United States' Food and Drug Administration (FDA).

- **Category A.** Well-controlled studies have failed to demonstrate that the medication presents a risk to the fetus in the first trimester, or in later trimesters. Examples of Category A substances include folic acid and levothyroxine (thyroid medication). The major point to know about Category A medication is that safety studies are conducted in humans, not animals.
- **Category B.** No adequate studies have been done in humans in this category. To be deemed safe, the medications given to animals must not result in malformations in their offspring. Category B medica-

tions include antibiotics like amoxicillin, ondansteron (Zofran) for nausea, and insulin used for diabetes.

- **Category C.** The medications in this category have demonstrated a risk for anomalies in animal studies. Again, no adequate controlled studies have been conducted in humans. When Category C medications are necessary during pregnancy, the potential benefits must outweigh the medicine's potential risks. This category also includes medications that have not had adequate animal or human studies. Medications include fluconazole (Dilfucan) for yeast infections, sertraline (Zoloft) and fluoxetine (Prozac) for depression and anxiety, and albuterol for asthma.
- **Category D.** Human studies have shown that when medication in this category was used by pregnant women, some babies were born with malformations attributed to the medicine. The prevailing thought is that in some cases this medication can be more of a benefit than a harm. Examples of medications in this category include paroxetine (Paxil), lithium for bipolar disorder, most chemotherapeutic agents, and most anti-anxiolytics like Ativan and Xanax.
- **Category X.** Human and animal studies have shown that mothers using this category of drug during pregnancy may have babies with problems related to the medication. Because there are no situations in which the risks outweigh benefits, these drugs should never be used by pregnant women. Examples are Accutane for acne and thalidomide, a sedative used to treat a specific cancer called multiple myeloma. It was used in the 1950s and 1960s as a medication for morning sickness.

12. After the birth of my baby, they will take him or her away and perform multiple painful tests.

Years ago, babies were taken to the hospital nursery for care after delivery. Consequently, mothers would have to go to visit their newborns. This separation caused anxiety and poor bonding between the mother and child. Today, with the development of labor-delivery-recovery-postpartum (LDRP) rooms, a patient now labors, delivers, and recovers in the same room along with her baby. Labor and delivery nurses will attend to mother and baby unless the delivery involves high-risk circumstances, in which case nursery staff will be called in to participate. Once the baby is born, and in most cases, after the mother has had time to bond and breastfeed, some tests will be performed. These tests can be performed in the delivery room and usually in front of the parents. Some of these tests will have obvious reasons, such as measuring and weighing the baby, while other tests may seem confusing to the parents. Let's look at the tests that will be performed after the delivery of your baby.

- **Length and weight.** The point at which this test is performed will vary from center to center and from nurse to nurse. Many mothers want to spend time bonding with the baby immediately after birth. Others will want to know the weight immediately and may not want to hold their baby until he or she has been cleaned. If you have particular desires, please let your delivering provider or nurse know your thoughts prior to the delivery.
- **Eyedrops.** Erythromycin drops are given to protect the baby's eyes from chlamydial infection, which, unfortunately, is all too common in our society. Chlamydia is the leading cause of neonatal conjunctivitis, which can lead to blindness. There are state laws governing the application of these drops, so you may want to become familiar with those laws or protocols. The eyedrops may make it a bit more difficult for your baby to see immediately after administration, but they will not burn or harm the baby.
- **Vitamin K injections.** Babies are not born with a complete set of clotting factors—the chemicals in the body that help us stop bleeding. During times when forceps and vacuum deliveries were more commonplace, vitamin K protected against the possible complication of bleeding in the brain when either of these delivery methods were used. Today, however, physicians use forceps less frequently, so vitamin K may not be needed. Again, vitamin K injections tend to be governed by state laws. Find out the laws in your state and make an informed decision.
- **PKU testing.** *Phenylketonuria* is a genetic disorder that is transmitted recessively. This means that if both parents are carriers of this trait, they have a 25 percent chance of giving birth to a child with this enzymatic disorder. Patients with PKU have a deficiency in an

enzyme that breaks down the amino acid phenylalanine, which is present in the American diet. Warnings now appear, for instance, on most cans of soda. Left untreated, this disease process can cause brain injury and mental retardation. The test is routinely performed anywhere from twelve to twenty-four hours after birth and is done via a small heel stick.

- **APGAR.** The APGAR test is named after the physician who described the system, Virginia Apgar, MD (1909–1974). Dr. Apgar, a pediatrician and anesthesiologist, devised the APGAR score as a means to assess fetal well-being immediately after birth.[18] The scoring system is done in five areas: **A**ppearance, **P**ulse, **G**rimace, **A**ctivity, and **R**espiration. Each category can have a score of 0 to 2 (see table below).

	Score of 0	Score of 1	Score of 2	Component of acronym
Skin color	blue all over	blue at extremities body pink (acrocyanosis)	no cyanosis body and extremities pink	**A**ppearance
Pulse rate	absent	<100	>100	**P**ulse
Reflex irritability	no response to stimulation	grimace/feeble cry when stimulated	sneeze/cough/ pulls away when stimulated	**G**rimace
Muscle tone	none	some flexion	active movement	**A**ctivity
Breathing	absent	weak or irregular	strong	**R**espiration

APGAR scoring system

This system of scoring is done at both one minute and five minutes of life; occasionally a ten-minute APGAR score will be performed if the first two are particularly bad and fetal resuscitation is required. The APGAR test is not used to determine if the baby will require resuscitation, but it can give pediatricians an idea about the state of the infant's brain function. Lower scores (less than 3) may be more common on the one-minute APGAR due to umbilical cord issues, such as a cord wrapped around the baby's neck. A lower score at one minute does not indicate a problem as long as the scores rise at five minutes and ten minutes. If, however, the scores remain low at the five-, ten-, and fifteen-minute marks, there may be some neurological damage.[19]

- **Universal Newborn Hearing Screening.** This test is called universal because all babies should be tested and can be tested before they leave the hospital. Hearing is essential for language, so it is necessary to determine whether there is any hearing loss in a newborn prior to language development. Currently the two types of testing are Otoacoustic Emissions (OAE) and the Auditory Brainstem Response (ABR). With OAE, earphones are placed in the ear and test results are determined by an echo recorded in the ear by a microphone. A baby with hearing loss will show a decreased or absent echo. During ABR, sounds are played into the baby's ears while skin detectors on the baby's head record the response of the auditory nerve. While up to 10 percent of babies fail their first hearing test, less than 1 percent will end up with permanent hearing loss. If babies fail their hearing tests, nursing staff and pediatricians will more than likely schedule follow-up testing one to two weeks after birth. Failures can occur for something as simple as debris in the ear canal or moving or crying during the test.

13. Breastfeeding will help with delivery of the placenta.

As we discussed earlier, there are three stages of the delivery process. During the third and final stage, the placenta is delivered. Normal deliveries take from zero to thirty minutes. In a majority of cases the placenta spontaneously separates from the uterine wall and needs no assistance. Does early breastfeeding help with delivery of the placenta? Recent studies show that breastfeeding within the first hour of life is essential for an increased rate of placental delivery and increased bonding of mother and infant.[20] We find, anecdotally, that by the time the baby begins actively breastfeeding, the majority of placentas have already been delivered. In most cases the placenta shears away from the uterus with the subsequent postpartum contractions. Signs of this placental separation include a gush of blood and lengthening of the umbilical cord.

A 2000 study classified different phases of the placental delivery as follows:

- **Latent phase.** The interval from the delivery of the infant to the beginning of uterine contractions that lead to placental separation.
- **Contraction phase.** Characterized by the uterine contractions at the placental site.
- **Detachment phase.** The placenta shears away from the uterus.
- **Expulsion phase.** The placenta and umbilical cord are delivered through the cervix and vagina.[21]

How then would early breastfeeding aid in the delivery of the placenta? Breastfeeding is primarily controlled by the hormones oxytocin and prolactin. When the infant suckles, there is a stimulant signal to the brain's hypothalamus to release oxytocin, which causes uterine contractions, and prolactin, which increases milk production. This oxytocin is the same oxytocin (Pitocin) administererd through an IV to stimulate labor contractions. Oxytocin also stimulates the lactiferous ducts to expel milk into the infant's mouth. Many women complain of cramping and pain after breastfeeding, commonly known as "after pains." These cramps result from oxytocin release and serve four purposes: expulsion of the placenta, contraction of the uterus to decrease postpartum bleeding, ejection of milk from the breast, and contractions to aid the uterus in returning to its pre-pregnancy size.

14. There is a 1-in-4 chance that I will have to have a cesarean section.

It is true that the cesarean section rate for *all* pregnancies is about 25 percent. The fact that this percentage represents all pregnancies is significant because it includes women who have had cesarean sections in the past and are electing to have a repeat C-section. So it is important for most women who have never had a child or have never had to have one by C-section to be informed of their chance of having a C-section. This means eliminating the number of elective repeat cesarean sections, which would be approximately 10 percent—a significant difference.

So why is the US national cesarean section rate 25 to 27 percent? We think there are a few reasons why: as one notable saying goes, "once a C-section, always a C-section." Some experts think that more and more women are asking for a first-time, purely elective cesarean section. Yet in a survey that asked 1,600 women who had undergone cesarean section why they had the surgery, only one person admitted that it was because of a personal desire.[22] This means that while women do request a primary C-section, meaning they have never had a C-section, the number is relatively insignificant. Perhaps there are more indications for C-sections and physicians are merely adjusting accordingly. The indications for a cesarean section are numerous, but there are some that might be more controlled by our current medical system than others. Data suggest, for example, that women who undergo induction of labor with a cervix that is not ripened (see Bishop's score) have a higher rate of C-section. Some people claim that the invasive nature of hospital care also contributes to the rising cesarean rate, although there are minimal data to support this.

Fifteen years ago, it was common for physicians to offer women an attempt at vaginal birth after cesarean section (VBAC). Today, women who desire a VBAC may not be given the choice. Physicians and hospitals are less eager to perform VBACs because of the small but substantial risk of uterine rupture.

Rates of uterine rupture during VBAC range from 0.02 percent to 9 percent, depending on the type of uterine incision.[23] Women who have a low transverse incision (side-to-side) have a rupture rate of 0.02 percent to 1.5 percent, while those with a classical incision on the uterus (up-and-down) have rates from 2 percent to 9 percent. In many cases of uterine rupture, the fetus will either die or be severely damaged by acute blood loss. When women learn there is an approximately 1 in 200 chance that their baby will be seriously injured during VBAC, many opt for the repeat cesarean section. The truth of the matter is that both physicians and mothers may be more cautious about performing VBAC deliveries simply because of this increased risk.

Women who desire a vaginal birth after cesarean section should also consider the reason for their cesarean section in the previous pregnancy. If a cesarean section was performed because the baby would not fit through the pelvis (cephalopelvic disproportion), this may indeed be the case in subsequent pregnancies. While some hospital statements show increased reimbursements for cesarean sections, some studies have shown that VBAC is actually more expensive.[24]

Obviously, the concern for cesarean section is real and with rates close to 30 percent there is a need to investigate and at least consider its possible etiologies. The decision to perform a cesarean section should not be taken lightly, as all surgery has inherent risks. The decision to proceed with cesarean delivery is a decision made between the patient and her health-care provider. In our experience, this decision is never made lightly, and we carefully consider the care of both mother and baby.

15. I cannot have a doula at my hospital delivery.

As mentioned previously, the word *doula* comes from ancient Greek, meaning "woman who serves." A doula can be of service during the antepartum, delivery, or postpartum period. To the best of our knowledge, no rules prohibit doulas from caring for women who deliver in hospitals. In our opinion, if the patient desires the aid of a doula, she should become a part of the patient's support team. We have attended many deliveries where a doula has been in attendance, and they have all been very pleasant experiences. A birth doula has her client's physical and emotional needs at heart. She will stay with the patient during labor and will help with communication between the woman and her healthcare team. The doula may also be present during the immediate postpartum period and can aid in breastfeeding and offering emotional support as well. We have also seen doulas help women with things such as caring for babies and helping with household duties in the prolonged postpartum period. In many cultures, new mothers are supported either by their mother or another woman close to them for many months after the baby is born. This seems common in other countries but very rare in our culture. The doula can provide care, comfort, and support in the crucial recovery period after delivery.

16. I will automatically receive an episiotomy.

An episiotomy is an incision through the lower part of the vagina into the perineal body, the perineal body being that portion of tissue between the vagina and the anus. The medical necessity for an episiotomy is to enlarge the vagina to aid in delivery of the fetus during the second stage of labor.

Medio-lateral episiotomy is at a 30- to 40-degree angle and is thought to result in less incidence of damage to the anal sphincter as well as providing more space for delivery. However, it is also considered to be more difficult to repair and is associated with increased postpartum pain and blood loss.

The most commonly performed episiotomy is the midline version, which is made at a 90-degree angle. Although the midline, also called a median episiotomy, is thought to have more incidence of injury to the anal sphincter (third degree) or the rectum (fourth degree), it is generally accepted as easier to repair and is associated with less pain with healing. In the 1920s, episiotomies were routinely performed because they were thought to reduce neonatal trauma and prevent urinary incontinence, the leaking of urine from the bladder unintentionally after childbirth or later in life. They were also thought to prevent pelvic organ prolapse, which is when the bladder, rectum, and/or uterus fall into the vagina and even outside of the vagina. In 2000, only 33 percent of deliveries involved episiotomy.[25] The reason most physicians no longer perform episiotomies is because median incisions do have an increased risk of anal injury and it has not been seen to reduce the risk of urinary incontinence or prolapse later in life.

A common myth among women is that an episiotomy will have more postpartum pain than a laceration that occurs naturally during labor. The American College of Obstetrics and Gynecology published a practice bulletin called "Episiotomy: Clinical Management Guidelines for Obstetricians-Gynecologists," in which it was reported that when comparing a laceration to episiotomies with the same depth, women complained of similar levels of postpartum pain; return to sexual activity was also the same between both groups. The report concluded that there is no evidence-based indication for the routine use of episiotomy. This is not to say that episiotomy is not indicated, it is just not considered a routine procedure. We recommend you discuss this procedure with your provider. Specifically, ask your provider if he or she performs this procedure on a routine basis. You should also remember this when you are admitted to the hospital and presented with consent forms that state that the patient understands that an episiotomy may be performed if indicated by the provider.

So, the delivery is the summation of the entire pregnancy. Some experiences are going to be good, and some are going to be not so good. However, either way, rest assured they will be memorable and worth talking about for years and years to come. This birthing process is rich in superstitions and myths, and that's what makes it so interesting. Our main advice is to plan for everything and have no expectations. Whatever your expectations are, your experience is sure to exceed them.

Notes

1 http://serendip.brynmawr.edu/biology/b103/f01/web1/fallon.html (accessed January 18, 2009).

2. R. Seropian and B. M. Reynolds, "Wound Infections after Preoperative Depilatory versus Razor Preparation," *American Journal of Surgery* 121 (1971): 251; H. W. Hamilton and K. R. Hamilton, "Preoperative Hair Removal," *Canadian Journal of Surgery* 20 (1977): 269; J. Tkach, A. M. Shannon, and R. Beastrom, "Pseudofolliculitis Due to Preoperative Shaving," *Association of Operating Room Nurses* 30 (1979): 881.

3. L. Reveiz, H. Gaitan, and L. G. Cuervo, "Enemas during Labour," *Cochrane Database of Systematic Reviews* 4, no. CD000330 (2007). DOI: 10.1002/14651858. CD000330.pub2.

4. A. J. Gagnon and J. Sandall, "Individual or Group Antenatal Education for Childbirth or Parenthood, or Both," *Cochrane Database of Systematic Reviews* 3, no. CD002869 (2007). DOI: 10.1002/14651858.CD002869.pub2.

5. I. W. Kelly et al., "The Moon Was Full and Nothing Happened: A Review of Studies on the Moon and Human Behavior and Human Belief," in *Skeptical Inquirer*, 10 vols. (Amherst, NY: Prometheus Books, 1986), 10:129.

6. I. W. Kelly and R. Martens, "Lunar Phase and Birthrate: An Update," *Psychological Reports* 75 (1994): 507.

7. G. R. Hamilton and T. F. Baskett, "In the Arms of Morpheus: The Development of Morphine for Postoperative Pain Relief," *Canadian Journal of Anaesthesia* 47 (2000): 367.

8. Judith Lothian, "Listening to Mothers: Report of the First National U.S. Survey of Women's Childbearing Experiences," *Journal of Perinatal Education* 12, no. 1 (2003): vi.

9. E. D. Hodnett, "Pain and Women's Satisfaction with the Experience of Childbirth: A Systematic Review," *American Journal of Obstetrics & Gynecology* 186 (2002): S160.

10. L. M. Goetzl, "Obstetric Anesthesia and Analgesia: ACOG Practice Bulletin and Clinical Guidelines for Obstetricians-Gynecologists," *Obstetrics & Gynecology* 100 (2002): 177.

11. L. J. Mayberry, "Epidural Analgesia Side Effects, Co-Interventions, and Care of Women during Childbirth: A Systematic Review," *American Journal of Obstetrics & Gynecology* 186 (2002): S81.

12. D. B. Scott and M. E. Tunstall, "Serious Complications Associated with Epidural/Spinal Blockade in Obstetrics," *International Journal of Obstetric Anesthesia* 4 (1995): 133.

13. http://www.lamaze.org/AboutLamaze/MissionandVision/Lamaze PhilosophyofBirth/tabid/378/Default.aspx (accessed January 21, 2009).

14. N. Lowe, "The Nature of Labor Pain," *American Journal of Obstetrics and Gynecology* 186 (2002): S16–S24.

15. L. L. Paine and D. D. Tinker, "The Effect of Maternal Bearing-Down Efforts on Arterial Umbilical Cord pH and Length of Second Stage of Labor," *Journal of Nurse Midwifery* 37 (1992): 61.

16. J. Roberts and L. Hanson, "Best Practices in Second-Stage Labor Care: Maternal Bearing-Down and Positioning," *Journal of Midwifery & Women's Health* 52 (2007): 238.

17. K. Eddleman, "Pregnancy Loss Rates after Midtrimester Amniocentesis," *Obstetrics & Gynecology* 108 (2006): 1067.

18. Virginia Apgar, "A Proposal for a New Method of Evaluation of the Newborn Infant," *Current Research in Anesthesia and Analgesia* 32 (1953): 260.

19. B. M. Casey et al., "The Continuing Value of the APGAR Score for the Assessment of Newborn Infants," *New England Journal of Medicine* 344 (2001): 467.

20. B. Dilek et al., "Does Early Breastfeeding Decrease the Duration of the Third-Stage of Labor and Enhance the Infant-Mother Interaction?" *Journal of Turkish German Gynecologic Association* 5 (2004): 208.

21. M. Krapp et al., "Gray Scale and Color Doppler Sonography in the Third Stage of Labor for Early Detection of Failed Placental Separation," *Ultrasound in Obstetrics and Gynecology* 15 (2000): 138.

22. http://www.childbirthconnection.org/article.asp?ck=10456 (accessed January 25, 2008).

23. http://www.mayoclinic.com/health/vbac/VB99999/PAGE=VB00007 (accessed January 25, 2008).

24. C. R. Pearman, "Does a Policy of Offering VBAC Really Save Money?" poster session presented at the annual meeting of the American College of Obstetrician Gynecologists, Denver, CO, May 1996.

25. T. J. Repke, "Episiotomy: ACOG Practice Bulletin No. 71," *Obstetrics & Gynecology* 107, supplement (2006): 957.

Section Five

The Mythical Grab Bag
Placentas, Twins, and Culture

Chapter Ten

Placentas, Cords, and Cauls
Cutting the Cord on the Afterbirth

The placenta, or afterbirth, and the umbilical cord, which connects the fetus to the mother during pregnancy, are a mythological goldmine—rich in significance to cultures all over the world. From long ago Stone Age times to today, humans have honored and sometimes even worshipped these organic ties that bind mother to child, seeing a deeper meaning: the binding of child to ancestors and to the unseen spirit world from which all life emanates.

The fate of the afterbirth, the umbilical cord, and the caul are considered by many cultures to determine the fate of the person with whom they enter the world. The afterbirth is sometimes said to contain the soul essence of a person, to be his or her guardian spirit or spirit double or twin.

Until recently, placentas were given short shrift by the medical establishment. Some hospitals even sold them to companies that made dog food (we heard about this in medical school). You may have seen hair care products touting their placental ingredients; luckily, this is bovine placenta. Today, the power of the placenta is being reevaluated by parents as well as by science. This amazing organ's lure and lore continue to fascinate, and in today's global culture, practices like burying placentas with trees (birth trees) or ritually eating placentas (placentophagy) are experiencing a rebirth of their own.

179

Placenta Power

Although most Westerners cannot recall or do not know where their own placentas ended up, many people from other parts of the world can tell you exactly where their placentas are. In fact, for many people from non-Western cultures (and some Western ones), knowing where the afterbirth is located is an important part of life and connection with family, community, and the world itself.

> We had recently moved to Tucson. A wonderful American Indian couple came into delivery while I was on call. The birth went beautifully, no complications, and mother and baby were doing very well just after birth. The baby was lying on the mother's tummy, and I was waiting for the placenta to deliver. The husband said, "Honey, remember, we have to take the placenta home." She looked up at me and said, "Yes, we want to take it home with us for a sacred ceremony." "Of course," I said, as though this was something I was familiar with. "I'll ask the nurses what the protocol is." However, I found out that there was no protocol and that the nurses had never been met with this request either. We did eventually find a way for the placenta to make it home with its rightful owners.

Let's first look at the placenta from a medical point of view.

The placenta is a blood-rich, spongy organ present in mammals, which connects to the uterine wall. The word comes from the Latin, meaning "flat cake." The German word for placenta is *Mutterkuchen*, and the Dutch word is *moederkoek*. Both words literally mean "mother-cake." The function of the placenta is to supply nutrients and oxygen from the mother's body to the fetus and to transfer waste products and carbon dioxide back from the fetus to the mother. It is also a hormonal powerhouse: producing progesterone, important to maintaining the pregnancy and somatomammotropin, which boosts glucose and lipids in the mother's blood as well as estrogen, relaxin, and beta human chorionic gonadotropin, which maintain the internal cushion of uterine lining for the fetus along with inhibiting other eggs from production and release.

The placenta also has an ingenious mechanism that cloaks it from the immune system of the mother. It stealthily secretes neurokinin B–containing phosphocholine molecules, which keep it under the mother's immune radar and allow it to carry on its functions without being attacked by white blood cells. The placenta contains high levels of prostaglandin, which stimulates involution (an inward curvature or penetration, or a shrinking or return to a former size) of the uterus, which has the function of cleaning out the uterus. The placenta also contains small amounts of oxytocin, which eases birth stress and causes the smooth muscles around the mammary cells to contract and eject milk. The placenta and amniotic fluid contain a molecule (POEF, placental opioid-enhancing factor) that modifies the activity of endogenous opioids in such a way that produces an enhancement of the natural reduction in pain that occurs shortly after and during delivery. This is not to say that the immediate postpartum period does not have its share of aches and pains, especially for those of you partaking in natural childbirth.

Eat It! Placentophagy

Most mammals eat the placenta after biting the umbilical cord off just after birth. Humans are one of the only mammals that do not sever the cord by biting. Some chimp species, genetically close to humans, also do not bite the cord. Eating the afterbirth, rich in nutrients, is said to help aid lactation and to ease postpartum depression.

Although not common in Western hospital births, eating the placenta (called *placentophagy*) is a practice that has been revived recently by parents seeking to connect with traditional folk beliefs and rituals of birth from times past. The media was abuzz when it was reported that actor Tom Cruise stated that he was going to ritually eat his wife Katie Holmes's placenta after the birth of their daughter, Suri (Cruise said later he never made the comment). British health writer Leslie Kenton recently chose to fry her son's afterbirth in onions and eat it on a British TV show called *TV Dinners*. The episode, widely watched and commented on, prompted twenty-one complaints to the Independent Television Commission—although British TV censors ruled that the program did not breach codes of taste and decency.

In the United States, where most placentas are discarded as medical waste, the practice of eating the afterbirth is not common. Women who want to take advantage of this practice sometimes have a hard time getting hosptials to release the tissue (considered by many medical institutions to be a hazardous bio waste). A recent lawsuit involved a mother, Anne Swanson, of Las Vegas, who sued the hospital where she had given birth for the possession of her placenta. When the judge ruled that she could have her afterbirth, Swanson said, "I'm obviously sad that it took a court case to get here, but I'm very excited that more women are actually going to be able to get their placentas if they want them."[1] The movement in this country for mothers to find healthy ways to ritually dispose of their placentas is in its infancy. Some hospitals may allow women to take their placentas home, just as they allow patients to claim their kidney stones and other discarded tissue or body parts, but this is on a request, case-by-case basis. In some instances, placentas are biopsied by doctors after birth to determine neonatal health issues. Check with your local hospital and attending physician if you are interested in taking home your own afterbirth. In many instances, any tissue that is removed or passed from a patient admitted to a United States hospital becomes the property of the hospital under the department of pathology.

The medical background behind the belief that consumption of the afterbirth eases postpartum depression and helps the mother to breastfeed may come from the fact that the placenta secretes a hormone called a corticotropin releasing hormone (CRH). This hormone tells the pituitary gland in the brain to secrete stress hormones. When the placenta delivers, there is a theoretic decrease in that hormone, which, according to some research, is thought to be at least partially responsible for postpartum depression. We have also discussed the question as to whether or not CRH plays a role in preterm labor, so there's a possibility that eating the placenta is one way to replete those hormones. However, because this has not been studied, we can't say that there might not be other harmful effects from this practice. So, from a medical standpoint, we cannot recommend eating your baby's placenta for dinner until more research is on the table.

> Neither of us has ever been asked about eating a placenta, and it is not something we spend much time thinking about. We can think of a few cases in which families wanted to have the placenta in order to take it home. In one case the hospital would not release the placenta at the time of delivery for whatever reason, so the patient and her family asked if they could at least dip their fingers in the placenta and wipe a small

streak of blood across their foreheads. It was okay by me, once I informed them of the potential for infectious materials and things of that nature. Each member of the family then dipped their fingers into the maternal side* of the placenta and smeared a line of blood across their foreheads. They also repeated this practice with the baby and new mother. It reminded me of the Catholic practice of smearing an ash crucifix on the forehead on Ash Wednesday—another way of exemplifying your beliefs and making an obvious mark to others that you are part of a particular belief system. In the case of the placenta, the smearing of blood marked the family members as part of a clan and welcomed the newest member, but instead of being a reminder of their mortality, this was an expression of birth and the power of familial bloodlines. I was not asked to participate in this ceremony not out of disrespect but because I was not part of this family's bloodline. This was one of the more truly powerful rituals I have seen, and the symbolic and concrete power was awesome.

Placentas in Chinese and Traditional Medicine

Traditional Chinese medicine has long revered the placenta as a healing organ with an aura of power and mystique—so much so that in China there is a black market for placentas, which are then served as special dishes in restaurants. This practice is illegal, however.

In Chinese medicine, the placenta is called *zi he che* and is considered a "valuable material" capable of treating lung disease and other ailments. If you refer back to the description of the placental physiology, you will see that the placenta carries blood and nutrients to the baby and carries away the baby's waste products. This is basically the description of a giant lung, as our lungs supply oxygen to the body while exhalation delivers our waste products into the air around us. It makes sense that Chinese medicine views the placenta as being capable of treating lung disease. In that type of homeopathic approach, an ailing lung would be treated with similar tissue.

"Placentas are dried and powdered and used as an effective medicine to enhance the functions of the kidney and to treat asthma," says Cai Gan, chief director of the Chinese Medicine Department of Shuguang Hospital.[2]

---

*This is the portion that is attached to the uterus and has a spongy consistency. The fetal side is where the umbilical cord attaches and is lined by the membranes; this side is shiny and smooth.

The perception of placenta as a Chinese medicinal cure-all has led to an illegal trade in the material and a response from the Chinese government. In China's Heilongjiang Province, for instance, the Ministry of Health has affirmed that placentas remain the property of the women who deliver them.[3]

So far, only the Shanghai Institute of Biological Products (SIBP) has been certified as a designated unit for collecting placentas from hospitals. According to the local *News Times*, SIBP paid hospitals 5 yuan (US¢60) for each placenta as a "service charge" (hospitals provide refrigerators to keep the placentas and pay for the electricity required).

Sources with SIBP said it was expensive to process placentas into medical preparations, as the process involves more than twenty different procedures. One kilogram of placenta powder sells for about 400 to 600 yuan (US$48 to 72) on the market.

In the United States there is a small minority of midwives and other advocates who believe in drying placentas and encapsulating them as medicine for postpartum depression, a practice the FDA has yet to recognize as valid. Again, we prefer to err on the side of caution. Placental material may carry HIV and other infectious agents and if not kept at optimal conditions, it may grow and spread germs that could be fatal if ingested. The extra nutrition in placental material that is thought to cure depression and help lactation can be ingested in the form of vitamins or other medically sound supplements. There is a growing contingency of individuals who are consuming the afterbirth because they feel it helps with the mother's nutrition and potentially with postpartum depression. However, most people living in the United States do not need to eat the placenta for nutrition because they have a grocery store down the street and in many cases a farmer's market that sells fresh fruits and vegetables. Members of societies who do eat placentas are more than likely doing so because of ritual or because there may not be an abundant food supply, and with the loss of blood and breastfeeding, the placenta may be the best thing available for the mother to eat. One of our patients claimed, "If it's good enough for a lion, then it's good enough for me." Lionesses typically have two to three cubs at once, they do not have a reliable food source, they are purely carnivorous, and the mother's nutrition is a life-or-death matter for her babies. One last thing about lions: they also occasionally eat their young.

Lotus Birth: Leaving Nature Intact

Some cultures (aboriginal tribes in Australia and the Balinese) believe in allowing the afterbirth and umbilical cord to fall off on their own. Some sects of Christians and Jews believe this practice echoes the Bible in describing the prophet Ezekiel: "As for your birth, the day you were born your navel cord was not cut." Some Buddhists believe that Gautama Buddha was born with the cord and placenta intact and was not separated from them until a time of his own choosing. Today, people are calling this process Lotus birth or Umbilical Nonseverance, and it is practiced by some birthing centers as well as by some home birthing facilitators. It is not a common practice in most American hospitals.

The process relies on presumed changes that produce a natural internal clamping of the cord vessels within ten to twenty minutes postpartum. The umbilical cord then dries to a sinew and naturally detaches from the umbilicus. Detachment generally occurs two to three days after birth.

For Full Nonseverance/Lotus births, excess fluids are wiped off the placenta and it is kept in an open bowl or wrapped in a cloth, in proximity to the mother and child. The cloths used to wrap the placenta or cover a bowl must allow air through, so that the placenta can begin to dry out. Sea salt and essential oils are often applied to the placenta to help dry it out.

Proponents of the method say it can prevent breastfeeding jaundice and loss of healthy birth weight, although there have been no proven medical studies on these claims. The reason most modern hospitals do not offer the procedure is in part because of medical conventions and protocols and in part because of the health of the infant. If the cord is not severed and the usual procedures are not carried out, there is a risk that, should a medical problem arise, the doctor or nurses may not have enough information to find and correct it. This would not be a concern when the birth is normal and everything is working smoothly, but it is common medical practice to first rule out what may be going wrong. We believe that although the "non-invasive, natural" idea behind Lotus birth is compelling, in many cases, it is safer to cut the cord and examine mother and newborn thoroughly after birth.

While the natural detachment of cord and placenta would be ideal for the emotional and physical bonding of baby and mother, the reality in a hospital setting is that the baby and mother at times require separation sooner for medical safety. Most placentas will detach naturally within thirty minutes, and the vessels in the umbilical cord will stop pulsing spontaneously after about twenty minutes. So, to leave the baby, cord, and placenta unit intact after that *may* invite more problems than it can prevent. The Lotus birth concept may have originated from the need to prevent infection of the umbilical cord—a need that no longer exists in our developed nation.

Again, there are no medical studies on this method, so it is difficult for us to recommend it. More important, we would say, there is no medical reason to cut and clamp the cord immediately unless there is a problem with either mother or baby. In the medical setting we are there to provide care to both patients, mother and baby. If all is well, there is no reason to intervene in the natural process. However, it seems there is no compelling reason that we know of at this point to prolong the process past the normal thirty minutes, and in fact, at that point, it could be unsafe for the mother to have the placenta remain longer.

Most placentas detach by that point naturally, and if they have not, there is a high likelihood that there is a placental abnormality, such as *placenta accreta*, which means the placenta has grown into the uterus and will not detach. If this happens, there is the potential for severe hemorrhaging, leading to an eventual hysterectomy and possibly even death.

Our "bible" for obstetrics states: "The timing of cord clamping should be dictated by convenience and is usually performed immediately after delivery. Although transfer of blood from the placenta to the fetus can continue for up to 3 minutes after birth, the volume of transfusion that results from delayed cord clamping is not clinically significant in most cases. After delivery, the infant should be held securely or placed on the mother's abdomen and wiped dry, while any mucus remaining in the airway is suctioned."[4]

Another ritual involves the father cutting the umbilical cord after the baby is born. If the husband or partner is too queasy, then another relative, often one of the grandmothers, will usually step in to do the honors. It is difficult to ascertain when this ritual started in our culture. We have come a long way since the 1950s, when men weren't even allowed in the delivery rooms but were instead banished to the waiting room where they smoked cigarettes vigorously and paced the room. Regardless of when or how this ritual began, having Dad cut the cord is a great way for him to be a part of the process.

Stone Children

Another aspect of the placenta we find fascinating is its ability to cling and grow—even in the most unlikely of environments. In very rare instances when the placenta attaches itself outside the womb during an ectopic abdominal pregnancy, the fetus dies and is then calcified on the outside, protecting the mother's body from the dead tissue and preventing infection. This is called lithopedia (from the Greek meaning "stone child").

World culture is full of tales of stone children—they often figure in folk and fairy tales. The true story is even more fascinating than the fairy tales. The condition was first described by Greek physician Albucasis in the tenth century CE. The earliest lithopedion was found in an excavation dated to 1100 BCE. Stone babies can sometimes go undiagnosed for decades. The oldest reported case is of a ninety-four-year-old woman whose stone baby had been inside her for over sixty years.

The Discovery Health Channel recently reported the story of a seventy-five-year-old woman who carried a stone child in her body for forty-six years until it compromised her health. She ultimately had it removed, and doctors said that had her body not retained and calcified the child, she may have died during a difficult procedure to remove the dead fetus, as medical expertise in 1955 for those procedures was limited. If this pregnancy had been abdominal* and attached to the intestines or abdominal wall rather than the uterus, and if the placenta had detached, there would have been a massive loss of blood and essential tissues. This type of pregnancy, by walling itself off and then calcifying the fetus, is protecting the life of its host, the mother.

Just like in a fairy tale, the stone baby had saved the woman's life.

Birth Trees and Other Afterbirth Rituals

As we have seen, the afterbirth is considered by many cultures to be a vessel of power and meaning. Just several years ago, many hospitals in the United States and abroad regularly sold placentas to medical firms for use

---

*In most cases the fertilized egg will find its way into the fallopian tube and uterus, where it eventually implants. Tubal pregnancies are those in which the fertilized egg implants in the fallopian tubes. In an abdominal pregnancy, the fertilized egg never makes it into the fallopian tube and in its quest for survival, it may implant on a vascular surface like the ovary or intestinal blood supply.

in medicines such as crèmes for burns and pills for the rare genetic disorder Gaucher's disease.[5] Today, as the placenta's cultural significance is recognized by more and more hospitals and legal entities, the sale of placentas by hospitals is declining. But it's not just because of placenta mythology. Britain has become the first EC country to ban the collection of human placentas because of new regulations about screening blood products to avoid HIV infection. There are currently no universal standards for placenta disposal. New mothers should ask their admitting hospitals about placenta procedures, as standards may vary.

Let's take a look at some of the cultural myths and legends about placentas.

The Placenta as Powerful Twin

From ancient times to today, the organ that feeds and nourishes the fetus while in his mother's womb has been revered, sometimes as a twin of the child and sometimes as an arbiter of the child's fate.

In ancient Egypt, the placenta of the Pharaoh was considered his twin and was carried into battle on a long stick. It's not surprising that other modern-day African cultures still have the same time-honored belief. In Central Africa, the Baganda believe that the afterbirth is the exact twin of the born child. It is put in a pot and buried under a plantain tree. The tree is watched carefully lest anyone eat from it and scare the twin spirit away. It is also thought that if animals eat from the tree, the human child may take on attributes of those animals.

The Cree Indians tell the story of the Bead Spitter and Thrown Away, in which a father watches the spirit of his son's placenta turn into a twin and play with his real child. Ultimately, the spirit becomes a real boy—an exact twin of his human child, whose fate is irrevocably intertwined with his twin's. Sumatran Bataks hold the belief that everyone has two guardian spirits—one lives in the seed of germination at birth and one lives in the afterbirth. Many Asian and aboriginal people believe that a placenta harbors powerful magic and must be buried in a special place, beneath a growing tree known forever to the family, so that the welfare of the growing child may be maintained. Even today in our American hospitals, some families, adhering to their ancestral beliefs, ask for the placenta so that they may bury it after the child is born.

Placenta Trees

The practice of burying a placenta beneath a tree so that the spirit of the child intertwines with the spirit of the growing tree is one that is honored in many cultures, from aboriginal Australia to Siberia. Today's modern world, which is in many ways frozen to the lore and legends of the past, is suddenly warming to the idea of placenta trees in more and more public ways.

Actor Matthew McConaughey and singer Rod Stewart have announced plans to the press to bury their children's placentas with trees.

McConaughey told Dr. Sanjay Gupta of the CNN medical show *House Call*:

> When I was in Australia, they had a placenta tree that was on the river... and all the placentas of all that tribe, all that clan—whatever aboriginal tribe that was—all the placentas went under that one tree.
>
> It was this huge behemoth of just health and strength. This tree was just growing taller and stronger above the rest of Mother Nature around it. It was gorgeous.
>
> That's fertile ground, so to speak. So we're gonna plant. It's gonna be in the orchards and it's gonna bear some wonderful fruit.[6]

Rod Stewart and his wife, Penny, are two other celebrities smitten by the placenta tree concept. Penny told her story to Britain's *Hello* magazine:

> We brought the placenta home and put it in the freezer so we could bury it later. When Rod's children Renee and Liam came over from Los Angeles, after lunch and before it got dark, we had a little ceremony. We doused the placenta in tea tree oil and placed it in a hole we'd dug in the garden.
>
> I said a few words like, "This is for our little Alistair. May he have a long and healthy life." Rod then passed a spade to Liam, who shoveled in some earth. Then we all took turns. We all jumped on the top and flattened the ground. It was a resting place for it.

This really does sound like a lovely ceremony, and it is wonderful to see the family participating in this type of ceremony as a way of initiating their newest family member. We live in Arizona, and the ground is so hard it is often impossible to dig. I am also not sure if this is something we would have to clear with our homeowners association.

Penny added, "My mum bought us a walnut tree and we thought it would be nice to bury it together."[7]

TV's *Baywatch* actor David Charvet, who is Tunisian and French, was recently seen coming back from the hospital with a box marked "placenta," allegedly to bury the organ in his own special tree garden.[8]

We can't comment on the spiritual effectiveness of these rituals, as they are a personal choice, but we do hope that you will follow the health guidelines of your care provider. If you are planning your own placenta tree ritual, we urge you to speak to your admitting hospital administrator or ob-gyn first. If your hospital allows patients to take home their placenta, you must follow their instructions about storage (freezing is usually necessary to prevent germs from growing and spreading) and disposal. The placenta is not considered human remains, and so it is legal to bury it, but in some cases your care provider may need to biopsy the organ after birth. If HIV or other infectious agents are present, it is against public safety regulations to bring it home and bury it. So do your own ancestral research and make your decision about disposing of your placenta in a *safe* as well as meaningful manner.

The Caul of the Wild

The caul (pronounced *call*) is another organ of birth rich in legend, lore, and meaning. Napoleon, Lord Byron, New Orleans "Voodoo Queen" Marie Laveau, and Liberace were all born with a caul. To be "born in a caul" is to be born with the head covered by the amnion or within an intact, unruptured amniotic sac. According to healthlink.mcw.edu, Dwight Cruikshank MD, professor and chairman of obstetrics and gynecology at the Medical College of Wisconsin, states that being born with, or in, a caul is rare, probably occurring in fewer than 1 in 1,000 births. He has seen fewer than ten babies born with a caul throughout his career.

We have seen this phenomenon only a few times, and although it is a natural process (it doesn't endanger the mother or baby in any way), it is a strange sight—the baby's face moving beneath the opalescent, wet tissue. We can understand why this unusual occurrence made people of times past believe that something supernatural was at work.

In medieval times, being born with a caul was considered good luck, and babies born with it were said to be marked for greatness (Liberace's mother would probably agree!). They were also said to have second sight and, according to some cultures, to be vampires (something said by various detractors about Lord Byron, who wrote one of the world's first vampire novels). In olden times a midwife would rub a sheet of paper across the encauled baby's head and face, pressing the tissue into the paper. The paper was then kept as an heirloom and sometimes sold to sailors who believed that the dried caul was a sure protection against drowning. Lord Byron's mother sold his caul to a sailor who took the treasured object with him on his next voyage. The ship was wrecked and the sailor promptly drowned. It is easy to understand the superstition of the caul bringing good luck to sailors if you look at the fact that if the caul was over the baby's face, it might seem like it had been protecting the baby from drowning by covering its mouth.

One of the most famous descriptions of a caul is in Charles Dickens's *David Copperfield.*

> I was born with a caul, which was advertised for sale, in the newspapers, at the low price of fifteen was withdrawn at a dead loss ... and ten years afterwards, the caul was put up in a raffle down in our part of the country, to fifty members at half-a-crown a head, the winner to spend five shillings. I was present myself, and I remember to have felt quite uncomfortable and confused, at a part of myself being disposed of in that way. The caul was won, I recollect, by an old lady with a hand-basket.... It is a fact which will be long remembered as remarkable down there, that she was never drowned, but died triumphantly in bed, at ninety-two.[9]

In Iceland, where fairies and spirits are still very popular, a caul is said to be a spirit double of the person to whom it is attached. This double will serve the person, and the person will serve the caul spirit during sleep when he carries out errands in dreams. The caul will tell the person of his imminent demise, appearing to him in a state illustrative of the manner of the person's death.

In New Orleans, home of the famous encauled Voodoo Queen, Marie Laveau, it is believed that the encauled child will become a seer into the unknown; the caul is considered a powerful aid that parts the veils between the real and spirit worlds—something that Laveau would have agreed she could do. Even today, pregnant mothers will visit her grave near the

French Quarter, leave a gift, and rap on the grave three times to ask her blessing on their child.

There is no way to create an encauled condition, and since babies born with a caul are a rarity, it is doubtful that many mothers will have the opportunity to sell or enshrine theirs. In a normal hospital birth, being born with a caul is rare but is not a health hazard in any way—the child can breathe through it and the doctor will simply remove it. If your child happens to be born with one, you can choose to believe in the positive aspects of caul lore or ignore it as an old wives' tale—but remember: those old wives often knew a lot more than we give them credit for!

The Umbilical Cord: Contemplating Our Belly Buttons

The umbilical cord is the tie that binds us to our mothers and to the lore and culture of birth since time began. In placental mammals, the birth cord binds the embryo or fetus to the placenta. The umbilical vein supplies the fetus with oxygenated blood from the placenta. The umbilical arteries return the deoxygenated, nutrient-depleted blood. This is the opposite of the function of the veins and arteries in our bodies. The veins carry our metabolic waste to the lungs, and the lungs bring oxygen to the arteries that then deliver it to our cells.

When the cord is cut and tied, the result is a mark that stays with us for the rest of our lives—the navel. It is a mark we have in common with all mammals.

There are hundreds of legends and myths connected with umbilical cords and navels—some of them still being passed to new mothers today. Many cultures believe that even after it is gone, the belly button, the place where we were originally connected to our mothers, is a place of power. Famously, Gautama Buddha is pictured contemplating his belly button. The Balinese call their island "the navel of the world," and the Greeks also considered the sacred site of Delphi to be *oomphalos*, Greek for "navel"— also considered "the navel of the world." In Kundalini yoga, the navel is said to be the site where the human being draws power into all the other chakras (energy points).

Up to 25 percent of fetuses are born with the cord wrapped around their necks. Some people say that if a mother raises her arms before pregnancy, the baby will be born with the cord around its neck. When the baby is born with the cord around its neck, the doctor simply unwinds it at birth. The presence of the cord around the neck has nothing to do with any position a mother takes while pregnant.

Cord Blood

Although it is a source of great mythological significance, the navel/umbilical cord area is also the site of a great deal of physiological power—the power of the baby's umbilical cord blood.

Cord blood is up to 180 mL of blood from a newborn baby that is returned to the neonatal circulation if the umbilical cord is not prematurely clamped. In some obstetric and midwifery practices, physiological extended-delayed cord clamping protocol, as well as water birth, allows for the cord blood to pulse into the baby for five to twenty minutes after delivery. If the umbilical cord is not clamped, a physiological clamping occurs upon interaction with cold air, when the internal gelatinous substance, called Wharton's jelly, swells around the umbilical artery and veins.

Cord blood possesses pluripotent cells: cells that have the ability to develop into any kind of cell and thus the potential to regenerate tissue. If you had a child with leukemia who needed a bone marrow transfusion, that child could theoretically receive the blood of his sibling if you'd planned ahead and had the blood banked.

That's where cord blood banks come in.

A cord blood bank can be a private commercial enterprise or a public medical resource used to store umbilical cord blood for future use. While public cord blood banking is widely supported, private cord banking is controversial in both the medical and parenting community. Blood collected this way takes up to 180 mL from the neonate (sometimes up to half of the total blood volume), which is a highly controversial subject in perinatal medicine. Cord blood is rich in hematopoietic stem cells,* however.

The American Academy of Pediatrics 2007 Policy Statement on Cord Blood Banking states: "Physicians should be aware of the unsubstantiated claims of private cord blood banks made to future parents that promise to

---

*These cells can give rise to any of the blood cells in the body. They can differentiate into white blood cells, red blood cells, and those cells called platelets that aid in coagulation of blood.

insure infants or family members against serious illnesses in the future by use of the stem cells contained in cord blood."

Cord blood is stored by both public and private cord blood banks. Public cord blood banks store cord blood for the benefit of the general public, and most US banks coordinate matching cord blood to patients through the National Marrow Donor Program (NMDP). Private cord blood banks are for-profit organizations that store cord blood for the exclusive use of the donor or donor's relatives. Expectant parents who want to save or donate their baby's umbilical cord blood must make arrangements by the thirty-fourth week of pregnancy.

Public cord blood banking is supported by the medical community. However, private cord blood banking is generally not recommended unless there is a family history of specific genetic diseases. New parents have the option of storing their newborn's cord blood at a private cord blood bank or donating it to a public cord blood bank. The cost of private cord blood banking is approximately $2,000 for collection and approximately $125 per year for storage, as of 2007.

At the time of publication, research is inconclusive, but studies point to the fact that cord blood is more effective when used outside the genetic material of the same family—hence limiting the actual effectiveness of the cord blood bank.

Videos have been circulated of children with serious diseases making miraculous recoveries after cord blood infusion—something we are extremely dubious about. We personally have chosen not to bank our children's cord blood, although we know other doctors who have. We believe this powder keg topic is something that has to be discussed by every family individually.

Donation to a public cord blood bank is not possible everywhere, but availability is increasing. Several local cord blood banks across the United States are now accepting donations from within their own states. The cord blood bank will not charge the donor for the donation; the ob-gyn may still charge a collection fee, although many ob-gyns choose to donate their time.

Notes

1. Steve Friess, "Ingesting the Placenta: Is It Healthy for New Moms?" *USA Today,* July 19, 2007.

2. Ibid.

3. Ibid.

4. Steven G. Gabbe et al., *Obstetrics: Normal and Problem Pregnancies* (New York: Churchill Livingstone, 2007), p. 316.

5. http://www.independent.co.uk/arts-entertainment/health—a-placentas
-life-after-birth-in-some-cultures-it-has-long-been-revered-women-here-are
-now-discovering-new-uses-says-sarah-lonsdale-1367563.html (accessed April 4, 2009).

6. http://www.starpulse.com/news/index.php/2008/08/09/matthew
_mcconaughey_to_plant_placenta_tr (accessed April 2, 2009).

7. http://www.femalefirst.co.uk/celebrity/Rod+Stewart-7865.html (accessed March 30, 2009).

8. http://celebrity-babies.com/2007/01/11/placenta (accessed April 10, 2009).

9. Charles Dickens, *The Personal History of David Copperfield,* 2 vols. (New York: Doubleday & McClure Co., 1899), 1:2.

Chapter Eleven

Twin and
Multiple Gestation Myths
The Magical Mirror

In the mythology of birth and fertility, perhaps no phenomenon has as much power over the imagination as twin and multiple births. Feared, worshipped, longed-for, and warded off, the birth of twins and multiple births like triplets and more can still move people to awe.

Even though we have been obstetricians for many years, even we sometimes still catch our breath when we see multiples. There's something about them that makes people feel they are experiencing something transformative—a supernormal event.

As most of us who pay attention to public media can attest, multiple births are very much in vogue these days. When celebrities like Charlie Sheen or Brad Pitt and Angelina Jolie have twins, everyone oohs and ahs. The notoriety of "Octomom" Nadya Suleman, who gave birth to octuplets with the help of in vitro fertilization, has put the topic on the front page, and pros and cons are being debated at watercoolers and over picket fences all over the country.

But it's not just Octomom who is birthing what are being called "super twins" (more than two twins: triplets, quadruplets, etc.). Thanks to fertility drugs and the increase of an expectant mother's age at birth, the number of twins and "super twins" being born in the United States is on the rise.

197

Twenty years ago, there were 90,118 sets of twins born in the United States, 2,529 triplets, 229 quadruplets, and 40 sets of five or more babies. In 2006, the CDC recorded:

- Number of twin births: 137,085
- Number of triplet births: 6,118
- Number of quadruplet births: 355
- Number of quintuplets and other higher-order births: 67[1]

The increase in multiple births doesn't just reflect a jump in babies being conceived with the help of medical technology; it is also the result of efforts by some obstetricians to help women bring those high-risk multiple pregnancies to term despite the odds. This practice is coming to be known as "extreme obstetrics," and it is being leveled as a criticism of the doctor who treated Nadya Suleman, the infamous Octomom.

Suleman rose to international "stardom" of a sort when she gave birth to octuplets (eight live babies) in January 2009. This birth marked only the second time a full set of octuplets has been born alive in the United States, surpassing the previous worldwide survival rate for octuplets set by the Texas-based Chukwu family in 1998.

Suleman's octuplets were conceived through in vitro fertilization: the technique for conception of a human embryo outside the mother's body. Eggs are removed from the mother's ovaries and placed in special laboratory culture dishes (petri dishes); sperm from the father or donor are then added, or in many cases a sperm is injected directly into an ovum, a process known as intracytoplasmic sperm injection (ICSI). If fertilization is successful, a fertilized ovum (or several fertilized ova), after undergoing several cell divisions, is either transferred to the mother's or a surrogate mother's body for normal development in the uterus or frozen for later implantation.

In the case of Suleman, all six embryos implanted into her womb took hold. Two of the embryos split into twins, resulting in a total of eight embryos. When doctors saw five thriving fetuses and offered Suleman the option of selective reduction,* she declined. The live birth of all eight

---

*Selective reduction is a controversial procedure in which the number of fetal implants is reduced by injecting a chemical substance (feticide) into the chosen fetus, which then perishes. When this is done in the first trimester the mother will reabsorb the blighted fetus.

babies put the newly dubbed Octomom into the limelight—a place detractors said had been her goal all along.

Public opinion skewed against her, mostly because she already had six children (two were sets of twins) from previous in vitro fertilizations. The doctor who implanted the embryos is under ethical investigation in California.* Another cause of the public's anger was that Suleman was on public assistance at the time of all the births. Apart from the media circus that has resulted from this extreme story of multiple births, the fact remains that whenever multiples occur, people instinctively react with great emotion.

In every culture around the world, the presence of twins is an event—something that portends either good luck or disaster, and we'll talk about that later in the chapter. In some African tribes, twins were considered evil omens and killed. In other tribes they were lauded as great good luck and were given instant high status among tribal members.

Even in our own day, we have personally seen fathers of multiples in particular take a certain swaggering pride in their planting. It's almost as if the presence of multiples makes them feel as if they have a stronger sperm count, which is not the medical reality of the matter. The formation of twins and super twins is not a miracle, but it is a fascinating process and sometimes an unexpected one.

I can vividly remember one birth when I was a second-year resident working on labor and delivery at the University of Oklahoma Health Sciences Center. At that time, we didn't have labor, delivery, recovery, and postpartum (LDRP) rooms. We would labor moms in their room and then take them back to the operating room for the actual delivery process; this was done for vaginal and cesarean deliveries. This particular night I was supervising a family medicine resident, and it was his turn to take the patient back for delivery. The process was simple, take the patient back and push the red button if you needed anything (the red button being the emergency button that would ring up at the nurse's station). I wasn't expecting anything out of the ordinary and was writing a progress note when, like a bleeding lighthouse, the backroom emergency light wailed on.

---

*In February 2009, the American Society of Reproductive Medicine released information that it was investigating the practices of Suleman's physician, Dr. Michael Kamrava. The investigation was looking at whether or not Kamrava followed ASRM guidelines when he knowingly implanted Suleman with six embryos.

I ran to the back and found a beautiful baby in the warmer, pink and crying. Everything seemed in place until I noticed the look on the intern's face; it was somewhere between excitement and insanity. I walked over to him and whispered, "What's going on?" He raised his finger and pointed at the patient's vagina, "There's something still in there." I furrowed my eyes and pursed my lips looking at the umbilical cord hanging out of the vagina. "It's called a placenta," I said jokingly. He just stared and said again, "No, there's something else in there." With my curiosity growing I asked the patient if I could do a vaginal exam, and what I found stays with me to this day. My fingers bumped into another head, big, round, and hard. I looked up at the patient and said, "Ms. Smith, you're not quite done yet." She looked between her legs and said, "You mean the placenta isn't out yet?"

"No, ma'am, I mean you have another baby to deliver." Turns out Ms. Smith started her prenatal care only two weeks before her labor, and we didn't have time to get an ultrasound. This was the first and last time I have seen undiagnosed twins, and it is something I will remember always.

Before we delve into the myth-conceptions about twins and super twins, let's discuss the medical facts.

How Do Multiple Births Occur?

Multiple births happen when more than one fetus is carried to term in a single pregnancy. They occur in most animal species, although the term is mostly used to define species that are born to mammals whose birth is accompanied by a placenta.

Monozygotic (identical) twins form from a single fertilized egg, or zygote, that splits into two or more embryos. Each of those embryos carries the same genetic material. These babies are always the same sex and are physically identical, although their characters and personalities are often very distinct (more on that later!).

Dizygotic births are called fraternal, which means that there are multiple eggs that develop individually within one pregnancy. The result is siblings who are no more alike genetically than other siblings. Fraternal twins are far more common than identical twins. Human multiple births can occur either naturally (the woman ovulates multiple eggs or the fertilized egg splits into two) or as the result of infertility treatments such as IVF (several embryos are transferred to compensate for lower quality) or fertility drugs (which can cause multiple eggs to mature in one ovulatory cycle). Multiples called polyzygotic represent some combination of fraternal and identical siblings. A set of triplets, for instance, may be composed of identical twins from one egg and a third sibling from a second egg. High orders of multiple births (three or more offspring in one birth) may result in a combination of fraternal (genetically different) and identical (genetically identical) siblings. The latter are also called *super twins*. For example, a set of quadruplets may consist of two sets of identical twins; in such a case each child has one identical and two fraternal siblings.

Multiple siblings in humans are invariably born prior to forty weeks of gestation, the average length of pregnancy. Thirty-six weeks is about average for twin births, thirty-four weeks for triplets, and thirty-two weeks for quadruplets.* Much of the increase can probably be attributed to the impact of fertility treatments, such as in vitro fertilization. Younger patients who undergo treatment with fertility medication containing artificial follicle-stimulating hormone (FSH), followed by intrauterine insemination, are particularly at risk for multiple births of higher order.

Some factors appear to increase the likelihood that a woman will naturally conceive multiples. These factors include:

- **The mother's age.** Women over 35 are more likely to have multiples than younger women. The increase of births in women over 35 means more twins worldwide.
- **The mother's use of fertility drugs.** Approximately 35 percent of pregnancies arising through the use of fertility treatments such as IVF involve more than one child.
- **Heredity.** A history of multiple births on a woman's side of the family increases her chances of having a multiple pregnancy.
- **Race.** Women of African descent are the most likely to have multiple pregnancies.

---

*It should be stated that twins and other multiples mature approximately one week faster than singleton gestations due to the added stress they face in utero. Nature has a built-in mechanism for accelerated maturation in twins as if it knows they will deliver early. Girls also mature faster than boys, both in utero and after they are born. This may be an added advantage for females, who carry the responsibility for the existence of the human race.

- **Number of prior pregnancies.** Having more than one previous pregnancy, especially a multiple pregnancy, increases the chance of having a multiple pregnancy.

Both delayed childbearing and infertility drugs are the two major factors from this list that have been on the rise in the last couple of decades. Culturally, the occurrence of multiples doesn't seem as shocking or as unique as back in 1934, when the world's first and so far only set of verified identical quintuplets was born on May 28, 1934. Cecile, Marie, Annette, Emilie, and Yvonne Dionne of Ontario, Canada, are believed to have been born around twenty-eight weeks, and the combined weight of the quints was a mere fourteen pounds. They were put by an open stove to keep warm, and mothers from surrounding villages brought breast milk for them. Against all expectations, they survived their first weeks. The Dionne quints became wards of the Canadian state and were on every cover of every magazine for years. They were the first media instance of the "super twin" phenomenon.

Far from the days of the Dionne quints, most multiples are now brought to birth without complication, but there are some risks involved. The most immediate risk is preterm (or early) labor resulting in premature births. A typical single pregnancy lasts about forty weeks, but a twin pregnancy often lasts between thirty-five to thirty-seven weeks. Nearly half of all twins are born prematurely (before thirty-seven weeks), and the risk of having a premature delivery increases with higher-order multiples.

Premature babies also face some important health risks. Because the care of premature babies is so different from that of full-term infants, preemies are usually placed in a neonatal intensive care unit (NICU) after delivery. The risk of developing health problems increases with the degree of prematurity—babies born closer to their due date have a lower risk.

In addition to the possibility of premature births, other medical conditions that are more likely to occur during a multiple pregnancy include preeclampsia, gestational diabetes, placental problems, and fetal growth problems. Being part of a multiple birth can also be associated with long-term health problems in the infants. Developmental problems and cerebral palsy occur more commonly in twins than in single births, and there's a higher risk of long-lasting health problems with higher-order multiple births.

Interestingly, there is a high instance of postpartum depression associated with multiple births* (perhaps some of the reason why certain cultures considered them "unlucky"?). The journal *Pediatrics* reports in a recent study[2] that mothers of multiple births had 43 percent greater odds of having moderate or severe postpartum depressive symptoms compared with mothers of single babies. Mothers with multiple births in the study had twins or triplets, and no significant difference was found in postpartum depression rates between those groups. It may be attributable to the actual stress involved in caring and feeding of multiples. The authors of the study also suggested that the process of in vitro fertilization was a stressful one and could contribute to the higher numbers of recorded postpartum woes.

How to Know If You're Having Multiples

In the first trimester, the only way to determine whether you are carrying multiples is through visual confirmation via ultrasound. Other indications may include:

- **Weight gain and a larger than normal abdomen.** Yes, we have many patients who come to us hoping that their excessive weight gain is due to twins. Some of them have just been "eating for two" a little too enthusiastically. But in some cases, the expectant mother feels a larger than normal presence, and weight and abdomen shape are larger than normal.
- **Fetal movement.** Normal single pregnancies don't usually cause movement in the first trimester, although mothers of multiples may have this sensation.
- **Nausea and fatigue.** Both nausea and fatigue in the first trimester may be signs of multiple births. This can also mean a regular singleton pregnancy more often.

Even if you don't personally want to know the sex of the babies involved when your doctor performs an ultrasound to see them, it is advisable from

---

*Most of us with children can understand the amount of mental energy it takes to raise one child, let alone two or more. It would make sense that there would be a higher rate of mental health issues in mothers of multiple births postpartum, as they are exhausted and have little time for themselves.

a medical standpoint. Only dizygotic (fraternal) twins can be different sexes. If the doctor identifies both male and female babies, you will know that your children will be dizygotic (fraternal), ruling out complications of monozygotic multiples such as twin-to-twin tranfusion—a random abnormality that causes one identical twin to receive less than normal amounts of blood supply during pregnancy while the other receives too much. The babies share blood vessels in their placenta that cause an imbalance of blood flow and nutrients between them. The myth of the "good" and "bad" twin may have developed from people observing this phenomenon—one baby being large and healthy and taking the nutrients and blood from the other twin.*

Common Myths and Questions about Twins and Super Twins

Maybe it's because having twins and multiples seems like such a strange and miraculous event (as if birth could get more miraculous!), but the mythoscape for multiple births is vast. You might hear that twinning skips a generation or that when you have twins, one will be good and the other evil. Or that because identical twins shared a womb, they need to share clothes, toys, and even the same breast for breastfeeding. Let's go over some of the most common ones:

The majority of multiple births come from infertility treatments.

False. Although twinning does have a high occurrence where fertility drugs have been used, the majority of twins and multiple births occur naturally.

---

*In a sense robbing Peter to pay Paul. When these twins are born there is obviously one that is chubby and healthy looking while the other is thin and frail looking. This could give rise to the possibility of one being greedy and the other being needy or breeding the potential that they must be opposites; a balance like yin and yang.

All pregnant women think they are having multiples.

Partial Truth. The truth is in the shades-of-gray category here. We have many patients who think they are having multiples because of excessive weight gain, which is not the cause of the baby, or multiples, but too many raids on the refrigerator in the middle of the night. On the other hand pregnant women have been found to be able to identify the presence of multiples before doctors confirm them through ultrasound. This is most likely because of actual movement and real fetal weight. As we've said earlier in the chapter, the only way to tell for sure in the first trimester is through a visual ultrasound.

**You can't breastfeed multiples,
or if you breastfeed you must never use the bottle.**

False. You certainly can feed multiples by breast and you can certainly supplement this activity with bottle feeding. In fact, we have had patients trying so hard to keep up with multiples that they have fallen asleep with a baby suckling at each breast. There are some doctors who offer supplementation as an option, and there is a particularly strident faction of the "breastfeeding police" that insists upon breastfeeding as the sole option for multiples. We think this is propagated by people who have never had the burden of feeding two infants at the same time or, even worse, at different times. However, we are not pediatricians and do not claim to be lactation specialists.

There's a good twin and a bad twin in every pair.

False. Humanity likes to see things in pairs. Good and evil. Black and white. So it seems natural that twins would be perceived as corroborating the two-makes-one theory. Like the yin/yang, there have to be equal and opposable forces. The reality is that twins are two individuals, and all old Bette Davis movies to the contrary, there is no evidence that it is natural for twins to divide into the evil/good motif. Young twins experiment with the balance of their relationship—trading off being the "good" and the "naughty" ones.* You'll find that each one of your multiples has his or her

---

*Although once they hit the "terrible twos," you are going to have two naughty ones.

own distinct personality—no one more "good" or "evil" than the other. This probably has more to do with the way the children are raised as in the self-fulfilling prophecy. If you expect them to behave badly, then they are going to be a pain in the butt!

Twins and triplets share everything.

False. Even though they have shared a womb, multiples are not inclined or required to share anything else except their parents' love. Of course, each must develop a sense of ownership of their clothes, and some toys. Most twins have their own amniotic fluid and placenta, so they don't really share anything but space. Parents can help children identify their own individuality by not requiring them to share everything and wear those cute sets of matching clothes that only tend to confuse the parents in the case of identicals.

They are always born by C-section.

False. While there are risks associated with multiple births that make cesarean sections a safer option, not all multiples are born that way. Some obstetricians even have a lower C-section rate with twins than with single births. The chance of a C-section increases with the number of babies; yes, higher-order multiples such as quadruplets or quintuplets are almost always delivered in the operating room by C-section. But many doctors are at least willing to attempt a vaginal delivery if conditions are favorable for both babies in a twin birth. However, in this day and age of litigation, doctors are less likely to do vaginal births with twins unless they are both head down (vertex) and the labor progresses normally. If one of the twins is breech, then a cesarean section is almost always recommended, and if they are both breech, then it is always a cesarean section. A worst-case scenario is the "locked twin" syndrome during labor. If the first baby is breech and starts to deliver the legs, body, and finally the head, but the second twin is head down and they lock chins while still in the uterus, then you have a medical emergency; none of us want to have a medical emergency.

Twins have ESP.

False. This is also an idea that belongs more in the realm of fiction, TV, and films than in reality. Everyone has heard the story that twins can feel each other's pain, know from miles away when their sibling has died, and other instances where "telepathy" can be cited as the reason for their uncanny connection. However, many instances of these types of "knowing" also occur among people who are not twins. Perhaps it is simply an intuitive connection of people who have grown up together, in similar circumstances. There is no evidence to suggest that twins are more "psychic" than other types of people. Again, in this circumstance, image and myth is more prevalent than actual fact.

They look alike and no one can tell them apart.

False. Some twins *do* look alike. Some don't. But even identical twins with extremely similar physical attributes have subtle differences. Once you get to know multiples as individuals, you can distinguish them.

The Magic Mirror: Twins in Myth and Legend

As we've seen, twins evoke an almost universal feeling of awe. Sometimes that awe turns to fear and sometimes to veneration. In Africa, for instance, it is said that an invisible line bisecting Nigeria defines the pro and con twin camps.*

The Yoruba and Guinea coast tribes to the west define twins as good luck; the Ibo and Cameroon tribes take the opposite position—twins are regarded as arbiters of misfortune. The "Cult of the Twin" is a powerful one in Africa, and the veneration of *Hohovi*, or twin figure, has even been transplanted to the cult of *voudon*, or voodoo, in Haiti, Cuba, and Brazil. As

---

*The rate of twins in West Africa is about four times higher than the rest of the world. In this zone is a town with the highest twinning rate in the world. The town is called Igbo-Ora and is referred to as "Twin Town." Twins in this part of Nigeria are considered gifts from God. In the dietary chapter of this book we discuss the wild yam and how some believe this root can increase the rate of twinning as it induces hyperovulation in the woman. Cassava is an essential part of the Igbo-Ora diet, and the skins of this tuber possess a chemical that can also induce hyperovulation. Many of the residents of this area believe the high twinning rate is due to their traditions, while others credit it with destiny.

icons of fertility, twins are featured in Benin's Voodoo New Year ritual in which villagers pray for the success of the next harvest.

Cassava flour and palm oil are two staples of the West African diet. During ceremonies, they are mixed in a ceremonial gourd and poured slowly on the ground. Benin practitioners of *voudon* believe that twins are undying spirits and harbingers of fertility and goodness. In Yoruban practice, fests are organized for the whole community when twins are born. The power of twins to bring happiness, health, and prosperity has a double edge, however. This same power is also said to bring disaster and disease if the twins so desire, and so they are often placated with ritualistic offerings. The firstborn twin, whether a boy or a girl, is always called Taiwo, meaning "having the first taste of the world." The second is named Kehinde, meaning "arriving after the other." Although born first, Taiwo is considered as the younger twin. His senior, Kehinde, is supposed to send out his partner to see what the outside world looks like. As soon as Taiwo has given a signal by crying, Kehinde will follow. Kehinde is supposed to be more careful, more intelligent, and more reflective, while Taiwo is believed to be more curious and adventurous, but also more nonchalant.[3]

On the third day after the twins' birth, the parents are visited by the community's Ifa priest. The oracle is able to drive out any evil spirits threatening the twins. He dedicates them to the Orisha, or god of twins, Ibeji. The Ifa priest also communicates to the mother a series of instructions on how to treat her twins: which colors they should wear or avoid, which food is recommended or prohibited, which animals are dangerous for them—sort of like a spiritual midwife. The Ifa priest will also recommend ways to exorcise any evil spirits he may deem to be present in either of the twins.

The Yoruba are said to have the highest rate of twinning in the world.[4] They brought their beliefs with them over the seas during the Middle Passage, when they were taken as slaves to the New World. Their carved Ibeji figurines (statues of twins) were venerated and hidden from slave masters who surely would have destroyed them as evil "heathen" gods. The figures were tied in the mother's wrapper as she sang and danced to offer praise. The figure was caressed, offered food, anointed with oils, and spent the night on a mat in the mother's bedroom, wrapped in a cloth to keep it warm.

African American couples having twins may wish to display ancestral images of twins or even buy Yoruban art depicting the sacred twin motif—

a vivid reminder of the strength of their own ancestors and a cultural motif of the powerful and auspicious twin. Perhaps twins were venerated because of their high numbers in Yoruban society—or perhaps those statistics are partly due to the positive treatment accorded twins in that culture.

African culture is not the only one to have made twins an important image and auspicious sign. In traditional Western mythology (the Greco-Roman motifs), Castor and Pollux and Romulus and Remus were important figures.

In Greek myth, Castor and Pollux were brothers to Helen of Troy and Clytemnestra, wife of King Agamemnon. Castor excelled as a horseman and Pollux as a boxer. They were great warriors and were noted for their devotion to each other. In one version of the legend, after Castor was killed by Lynceus, Pollux—in accordance with the classical tradition that one of every set of twins is the son of a god and thus immortal—begged his father, Zeus, to allow his brother to share his immortality with him. Zeus arranged for the twins to divide their time evenly between Hades and Heaven, and in their honor he created the constellation Gemini—the famous astrological sign of the twins. They were widely regarded as patrons of mariners and are said to be responsible for St. Elmo's fire, the luminous discharge of electricity extending into the atmosphere from some projecting or elevated object. This phenomenon is usually observed (often during a snowstorm or a dust storm) as brushlike fiery jets extending from the tips of a ship's mast or spar, a wing, propeller, or other part of an aircraft, a steeple, a mountaintop, or even from blades of grass or horns of cattle. It has been said that the nimbus created from St. Elmo's fire is the light seen around the heads of saints—yet another association of something sacred being connected to twins.

Romulus and Remus are the traditional founders of Rome, appearing in famous brass sculptures as infants suckling at a wolf's teats. They were the twin sons of the vestal virgin Rhea Silvia and were fathered by Mars, the god of war. Since the vestals were supposed to remain virgins, this birth obviously caused some consternation among the gods, chief among them Vesta, or Hestia, the patroness of the vestals and goddess of the hearth. The twins' mother was buried alive for her sins, and the boys were cast adrift on the river Tiber but kept safe by the river deity, Tiberinus, who made the cradle catch in the roots of a fig tree (sound anything like Moses in the reeds?). Later, the twins were nursed by a wolf, Lupa—an act that may be responsible for our current phrase denoting bad upbringing: "raised by wolves." Romulus and Remus are preeminent among the famous feral children in mythology and fiction and although they came to doubtful endings (Romulus slew Remus* and became the sole king of Rome), their image as dual and powerful figures remained in the classical world as icons of power and portent.

Another familiar Greco-Roman twin pair is Apollo, the sun god, and Artemis/Diana, his twin sister, the goddess of the moon.

According to the mythology of Central America, the Aztecs used to kill one twin of a pair, believing that such an act prevented the parents from an early death. The remaining twin was supposed to have great supernatural power and could use these powers for evil as well as good. The Tarascan people believe that female twins cannot cook tamales or squash. They also believe, like many people around the world, that if a pregnant woman eats "paired" fruits like cherries, bananas, and so on, she will have twins.

One of our favorite myths involves the saints Cosmas and Damian (also spelled Kosmas and Damianos), twins and early Christian martyrs born in Arabia who practiced the art of healing in the seaport of Aegea (modern Ayas) in the Gulf of Issus, then in the Roman province of Syria. They took no money for their services, which led them to be nicknamed *anargyroi* (the silverless). They were also famed for grafting a Caucasian person's leg onto the stump of a young Ethiopian boy—one of the first successful limb transplants (if apocryphal). The twins were beheaded for their Christian faith and are now the patron saints of twins, doctors, and organ donations. You are also supposed to pray to them when seeking reasonable medical fees. The association of twins with health-giving powers is widespread in mythology, folklore, and religion. The Ashvins of the Rig-Veda, the classical Dioscuri, and the early Christian saints Cosmas and Damian are among the many examples of twins divinely empowered in the area of health and fertility. Along with healing, divine twins are often empowered with the ability to revive the dead; increase the fertility of humans, animals, and crops; influence the weather, predict the future, and ensure victory in battle.[5]

---

*This act highlights two important points. First, it shows a parallel to Cain and Abel, who were not twins but whose story included the power of sibling rivalry and the concepts of desire, greed, and jealousy. Second, it emphasizes the fact that because twins may look alike, one or both can develop a desire to be different.

The miracle of birth continues to be multiplied in people's minds when seeing double, triple, and more. Even in today's technological society, twins and multiples have the power to astonish us!

Famous Mythical Twins

Helen of Troy and Clytemnestra, twin sisters of Castor and Pollux

Romulus and Remus, mythical founders of Rome

Lava and Kusha, twins of Lord Rama and Sita

Apollo and Artemis, son and daughter of Zeus and Leto (Apollo is the god of the sun and Artemis is the goddess of the moon, hunting, and fertility)

Heracles and Iphicles (twins from different fathers)

Castor and Pollux, the Gemini twins, aka the Dioscuri

Famous People Who Have a Twin

Who knew that Ann B. Davis from *The Brady Bunch* had a twin? Or Montgomery Clift? Or racing car driver Mario Andretti? The following list just goes to show you that there is often much more to people than meets the eye—and in the case of the identical twins, a mirror image, in fact.

James Alexandrou, British actor (twin sister Antoinette)

Chad Allen, American actor (twin sister Charity)

Carl Anderson, American singer/actor (twin died as an infant)

Mario Andretti, Italian American racing driver (twin brother Aldo)

Kofi Annan, former United Nations secretary-general (twin sister Efua)

Lillian Asplund, last American survivor of the *Titanic* disaster (twin brother Carl Edgar died in the tragedy)

Conrad Bain, Canadian actor (twin brother Bonar)

Gracia Baur, German pop singer (identical twin sister Patricia)

Blaze Berdahl, American actress (twin sister Beau)

Josh Bernstein, American explorer and TV host (identical twin brother Andrew)

Nicholas Brendon, actor (twin brother Kelly)

Jim Broadbent, British actor (twin sister died at birth)

Gisele Bündchen, Brazilian supermodel (fraternal twin sister Patrícia)

Gabrielle Carteris, American actress (twin brother James)

Karen Cellini, actress from the TV series *Dynasty* (twin sister Kate)

Justin Chambers, American actor (twin brother Jason)

Keith Chegwin, British TV presenter and former actor (twin brother Jeff)

Gary Cherone, American musician (fraternal twin brother Greg)

Montgomery Clift, American actor (twin sister Roberta)

Carlo Colaiacovo, Canadian hockey player (brother Paulo)

Henry Cooper, British boxer (twin brother George)

Bucky Covington, *American Idol* finalist (identical twin brother Rocky)

Andrew Daddo, Australian actor (fraternal twin Jamie)

Ann B. Davis, actress on *The Brady Bunch* (twin sister Harriet)

Tanja Dexters, Miss Belgium 1998 (twin sister Mieke)

Philip K. Dick, American writer (twin sister Jane, died after birth)

Vin Diesel, American actor (fraternal twin brother Paul Vincent)

Duffy, Welsh soul singer (twin sister Katy)

Karen Elson, British supermodel (fraternal twin sister Kate)

John Elway, NFL quarterback (twin sister Jana)

Theo Epstein, general manager of the Boston Red Sox (twin brother Paul)

Mike Espy, former US secretary of agriculture (twin sister Michelle)

Joseph Fiennes, British actor (twin brother Jacob)

Max Gail, actor (twin sister Mary)

Andy Garcia, American actor (parasitic twin brother removed from Andy's shoulder; died soon after)

Eva Green, French actress (fraternal twin sister Joy)

Jerry Hall, American model and actress (twin sister Terry)

Linda Hamilton, American actress (identical twin sister Leslie played the "T-1000 Sarah" in *Terminator 2: Judgment Day*)

Victor Davis Hanson, American author (fraternal twin brother Alfred)

William Randolph Hearst, newspaper magnate (twin died as an infant)

Jon Heder, American actor (identical twin brother Daniel)

Marilu Henner, American actress (twin sister Crystal)

Jill Hennessy, Canadian actress (twin sister Jacqueline; both appeared in the movie *Dead Ringers*)

John Hensley, American actor (fraternal twin sister)

Ryan Howard, first baseman for the Philadelphia Phillies (twin brother Corey)

Matt Hughes, martial arts fighter (identical twin brother Mark)

Marlon Jackson, American singer (twin brother Brandon died at birth)

David Jason, British actor (twin brother Jason died at birth)

Chris Joannou, bass player for Australian rock band Silverchair (twin sister Louise)

Scarlett Johansson, American actress (twin brother Hunter)

Kim Junsu, Korean musician (twin brother Junho)

Jay Kay, British singer (twin brother died at birth)

Cory Kennedy, American Internet celebrity (fraternal twin sister Chris)

David Kohan, TV producer (twin brother Jono)

Ashton Kutcher, American actor (fraternal twin brother Michael)

Kate Lawler, winner of UK *Big Brother 3* reality show (twin sister Karen)

Gigi Leung, Chinese singer (twin brother Keith)

Liberace, impresario (twin died as an infant)

Tony Liberatore, AFL footballer with the Western Bulldogs (twin brother Fred)

Cory Lidle, former Major League Baseball player (twin brother Kevin)

Thad Luckinbill, soap opera actor (twin brother Trent)

John Maine, Major League Baseball pitcher (fraternal twin brother)

Shawn Marion, NBA basketball player (twin sister Shawnett)

Susie Maroney, Australian swimmer (fraternal twin Sean)

Kim Mathers, ex-wife of rapper Eminem (nonidentical twin Dawn)

Paul McDermott, Australian comedian (fraternal twin)

Victor A. McKusick, professor of genetics (twin brother Vincent was chief justice of the Maine superior court)

Naima Mora, winner of cycle 4 of *America's Next Top Model* (twin sister Nia)

Alanis Morissette, Canadian rock singer/songwriter (twin brother Wade)

Burt Munro, New Zealand motorcycle racer (twin sister died at birth)

Mandy Musgrave, American actress (identical twin sister Jamie)

Jason Orange, member of British boy band Take That (twin brother Justin)

Gaute Ormåsen, Norwegian singer (fraternal twin brother Hogne)

Parker Posey, American actress (twin brother Chris)

Elvis Presley (twin brother Jesse Garon died at birth)

Richard Quest, CNN anchor (twin sister Caroline)

Dack Rambo, American actor (twin brother Dirk)

Judy Reyes, American actress (twin sister Joselin)

Giovanni Ribisi, American actor (twin sister Marissa)

Marty Robbins, country music singer (twin sister Mamie)

Isabella Rossellini, Italian actress (twin sister Isotta Ingrid)

J. D. Roth, American actor (twin sister Heidi)

Judith Scott, artist (twin sister Joyce)

Teemu Selänne, Finnish hockey player (twin brother Paavo)

Sab Shimono, Japanese American actor (twin brother Jiro)

Lori Singer, American actress (twin brother Gregory)

Gabriela Spanic, Venezuelan actress (twin sister Daniela)

Katy Steele, lead singer of Australian rock band Little Birdy (twin brother Jake)

Curtis Strange, professional golfer (identical brother Allen)

Ed Sullivan, TV host (twin died as an infant)

Kiefer Sutherland, Canadian actor (twin sister Rachel)

Amanda Tapping, Canadian actress (twin brother Chris)

Jim Thorpe, American athlete (twin brother, Charlie)

Jon Tickle, participant on UK *Big Brother 4* (twin brother Edmund)

Garrett Tierney, American musician (identical twin brother Shaun)

Paul Tsongas, American politician (twin sister Thaleia)

Ronan Tynan, Irish opera singer (twin brother died as an infant)

Sarah Vowell, American author (twin sister Amy)

Shayne Ward, British pop singer (twin sister Emma)

Billy Dee Williams, American actor (twin sister Loretta)

Ricky Williams, American football player (twin sister Cassie)

Marvin Winans, gospel singer (twin brother Carvin)

Will Young, British singer (fraternal twin brother Rupert)

Notes

1. http://www.cdc.gov/nchs/data/nvsr/nvsr57/nvsr57_07.pdf (accessed April 14, 2009).

2. Yoonjoung Choi et al., "Multiple Births Are a Risk Factor for Postpartum Maternal Depressive Symptoms," *Pediatrics* 123, no. 4 (2009): 1147.

3. Fernand Leroy et al., "Yorba Customs and Beliefs Pertaining to Twins," *Twin Research* 5, no. 2 (2002): 132.

4. http://www.africanart.org/past/26/doubly_blessed_the_ibeji_twins_of _nigeria (accessed April 27, 2009).

5. Leon D. Hankoff, "Why the Healing Gods Are Twins," *Yale Journal of Biological Medicine* 50, no. 3 (1977): 307.

Chapter Twelve

The Navel of the World
Global Myths of Birth and Fertility

O ne of the most fascinating aspects of working as an obstetrician-gynecologist in the United States is the fact that so many of our patients come from different backgrounds. When an African American woman shares her thoughts and concerns and tells us some of the "myth-conceptions" that she heard from her grandmother, such as "If you dream of fish, someone is going to have a baby," we understand that many of these beliefs have probably lingered since the days of the Middle Passage, when people from many different African tribes were brought to these shores as slaves. The fish tale may come from the fact that one of the Yoruban fertility deities—Yemanya—is often seen as a woman with a fish tail. The first African Americans brought to this country were not allowed to keep anything but their beliefs, and those beliefs have held strong through the centuries.

When we work with Native American women, we are reminded that much of what they know about childbirth was learned from their culture and tribal elders. The same is true for Mexican Americans, Italians, Scots, Irish, Germans, and Nordic Americans, and so on. The rich tapestry of myth in every woman's background should be a source of pride and plea-sure—not anticipatory fear and doubt—which is one of the reasons we wrote this book. We wanted to separate the real medical facts from the stories, while letting some of stories stand on their own as testaments to the culture and imaginations of the people who used them to understand the world and the miraculous process of birth.

Pregnant women stand at the threshold of the past and the future. The myths and stories that have been passed down in their families are like umbilical cords binding them back to the past and connecting them to the new generation. Instead of scoffing at these stories from a medical perspective as being "old wives' tales," we think we should understand the medical truth while at the same time honoring the tales and their tellers.

Why Our Stories Matter

In this book, we have tried to explain the common myths about birth from a medical perspective. In this chapter, we want to explain what these myths say about us as people and how they illustrate the unique ways in which we are human. It has been said that the human race is the only one that makes up stories about itself. Often the stories that are told about childbirth bear a nugget of medical truth, sometimes one that, even today, we do not fully understand. There is an old wives' tale, for example, that says that if you have heartburn when you are pregnant, your baby will be hairy. Strange, yes? A recent study done at Johns Hopkins University found that of sixty-four women giving birth, the ones with the most heartburn gave birth to babies with more than average newborn hair.[1] No one knows why as yet, but this is an example of people noticing things about the world around them and then interpreting them to make sense of the experience.

Who Were the "Old Wives"?

Many of the stories that get handed down to us are called "old wives' tales." An old wives' tale or old wives' saw is a type of urban legend, similar to a proverb, which are generally passed down by the older women in a family to the younger generation. Such "tales" usually consist of superstition, folklore, or unverified claims with exaggerated and/or untrue details. Old wives' tales often concern pregnancy, puberty, and nutrition.

The use of the word *wife* in this phrase refers more to a *woman* than a *married woman.* This usage stems from Old English *wif* ("woman") and is akin to the German *weib,* also meaning "woman." This sense of the word is still used in Modern English in constructions such as *midwife* and *fishwife.* Most old wives' tales were originally intended to discourage unwanted behavior, usually in children, such as the familiar "If you frown, your face will freeze that way." Among the few tales with grains of truth, the veracity is likely coincidental, but it may stem from the power of observation and cause and effect, which was an early form of science itself.

The concept of old wives' tales is ancient. In the first century, the apostle Paul wrote to his young assistant Timothy, "But refuse profane and old wives' fables, and exercise thyself rather unto godliness."

The "old wives" who originally came up with the tales that you might hear during your pregnancy may have also been midwives and herbalists, the women who traditionally in old Europe brought babies into the world. These midwives knew their herbs and herb lore, as well as the legends of their people that surrounded what real science they did know. In many cases it was these women who were burnt or hanged during Europe's famous "burning times," the hunt for "witches," which resulted in the slaughter of millions of innocent people—most of them women and a good many of them "old wives." So when you hear the phrase "old wives," you might imagine your ancestors and the fact that these "old wives" were doing their best to understand the world around them through these "tales." These tales were not concocted to deliberately deceive people, but as science has proved or disproved, many of them can be put into a new category—as myth, not fact, but no less relevant for not being "factually" true.

Ancient Myths of Fertility and Childbirth

All cultures have a creation tale—a story to explain how the first birth occurred. The Judeo-Christian story is of Adam and Eve and the garden of Eden, found in the biblical book of Genesis. Earlier tales from that tradition involved a figure called Lilith, sometimes called "Adam's first wife," who was actually a Sumerian fertility goddess to whom people prayed on behalf of children, crops, and health. In later days the story mutated, and she became a specter who haunted Adam and his new wife and killed their children—she is the first vampire in legend. Perhaps this tale was devel-

oped to explain the sudden death of infants that happened much more frequently in the days before modern medicine. Today, the image and name
of Lilith is often used by feminists who wish to reclaim her identity as a
beneficent goddess of childbirth and fertility rather than of death.

In the Middle East, Hathor, the great Egyptian fertility and childbirth
goddess, is perhaps most familiar to us as the Christian Bible's "golden
cow." Hathor was worshipped throughout the Egyptian empire, particularly in areas that are close to modern-day Somalia and in the Sinai region,
where Moses and the tribes of Israel wandered after leaving Egypt. She is
often depicted as a golden cow.

Hathor was a powerful and important goddess, much like her sister
goddess, Isis. Both deities were important for women during childbirth.
They assisted mothers in bringing forth healthy children and helped
women fall in love and get pregnant. Isis is often seen as a mother with her
baby Horus on her lap—a progenitor of many Madonna and child statues.
One of her most interesting charms or attributes is the *tyet*, or Isis knot. It
looks like an ankh but has two loops that fall downward. Some Egyptolo-
gists believe that it represents the fallopian tubes. Egyptian women would
carry amulets of the *tyet* on their bodies to ensure a safe pregnancy.
Another great Egyptian goddess of birth was Tawret, the hippopotamus
goddess, patroness of midwives. Bes was a dwarf god who looked like a
newborn and helped the divine ladies ensure a healthy birth.

These goddesses were even worshipped in the Roman world. Today
you can see images of Hathor in Pompeii in rooms that would have been
used by women for childbirth and even in areas dedicated as brothels.

In Ephesus (modern-day Turkey), the mother goddess supreme was a
virgin known as Artemis or Diana, the virgin goddess of the moon. Her
temple in the Roman outpost of Ephesus was famous for its huge statue of
the goddess festooned with hundreds of breasts from which she fed the
world. It is said the Christians later claimed that Mary, mother of Jesus, died
in Ephesus. This claim was intended to usurp some of the devotion paid to
the virgin mother, Artemis, by redirecting it to another virgin mother, Mary.
Diana/Artemis was known by many names including Queen of Heaven; the
Great Goddess; Lunar Virgin; Mother of Animals; Lady of Wild Creatures;
the Huntress; Patroness of Childbirth, Nursing, and Healing.

The Greeks and the Romans had Venus/Aphrodite, who embodied
many of the attributes of Hathor. We know her as the goddess of love, but

she was also considered the goddess of fertility, especially in the islands of her origin.

Even today, on the island of Cyprus, where she is said to have been born, local women practice rituals connected with her ancient worship. It is said that if you bathe in the famous "pool of Aphrodite" on the island, you will have many children and stay beautiful for a long, long time: the ancient version of Botox.

Childbirth and Fertility Lore Today

Although the existence of fertility rituals and the ritualizing of childbirth is fading in today's modern world, there are still aspects of it that linger. Our current-day ritual of Groundhog Day comes from the Celtic Festival of Candlemass, or Imbolc, a fertility festival that occurred around the same time as Easter. This is another example of a pagan holiday of fertility that was Christianized but that retained the symbols of eggs and breeding rabbits. Traveling around the world you will still see many ancient symbols of fertility, such as standing stones, tikis, and sacred wells. If you ask the locals, they will tell you that modern-day women visit these sites in the hope that the ancient cures and fertility rites still work.

Recently, residents in Great Britain were furious when a famous fertility icon, the Cerne Abbas Giant, near the Dorset town of Cerne Abbas, was defaced by an advertiser who turned the icon into a representation of the popular animated TV character Homer Simpson in an advertising stunt. The giant is actually a chalk drawing etched into a hill. It is remarkable because of its giant erect phallus and the legend that if you walk "widdershins" (backward) around his circumference, you will become pregnant. Many women in the area still practice this ritual. The advertiser was taken to task for defacing this important icon—especially because the giant icon was roped off and unavailable for several days to the eager local fertility walkers.

African and African American

African fertility and birth rites and rituals are perhaps among the better-known practices in the world because of the beautiful artwork associated with them. As we've seen in a previous chapter, twins are special in most

African tribal culture, and Benin and Yoruba artwork in particular is full of images of twins, originally created as devotional objects or fertility charms.

In particular, the Yoruban culture of the Orishas (the gods) has traveled over the seas during the Middle Passage to mutate into New Orleans voodoo, Haitian *voudon*, and Cuban Santeria and is still very strong today.

The Yoruban roots of Orisha worship have taken hold around the world but are more tenuous in Nigeria, where they were born. Every year the Osun-Osogbo Sacred Grove Festival in Nigeria brings hundreds of pilgrims from around the world as well as in Nigeria, where the Orisha religion is foundering. The week-long ceremony of fertility is as old as Africa itself. During the festival, worshippers flock to the river where they float sacred objects and flowers and ask Osun, the goddess of the rivers and flowing things, for the blessing of children and fertility.

Recently, alcoholic drink Seaman's Schnapps has been brought in as an "official sponsor" of the fertility festival—something that locals say will drive out the gods from the grove, along with the Europeans, who are increasingly coming to view the event as an international party event, much like Mardi Gras in New Orleans, which also has its roots in fertility festivals.[2] The Seaman's company bills itself as "the number one devotional drink" in billboard advertisements. Alcohol is traditionally used to invoke the goddess at the river and to offer her and her fellow gods a sacrifice. But this new commercialization of the ancient rite may ultimately drive away the "sacredness" of the site. When tourism and crowds come in, the gods may depart.

Another example of a sacred site in Africa is Victoria Falls—the spectacular waterfall between the countries of Zimbabwe and Zambia. The local river god Nyaminyami is said to have been parted from his wife when construction was started on a dam that was to create the new Lake Kariba. Many construction workers and animals lost their lives in the construction of the dam, which locals saw as a manifestation of the god's anger at losing his wife. Every year, the local Tonga people have a festival honoring the god, one of whose attributes is to bestow food and fertility to his people. Recently, at the falls, a new helicopter service was started for tourists to see the wonder of the falls close up. Local medicine men say that this is the final straw and that the god will now depart from the falls and go away forever.[3] If fertility rates drop too, we may look to science and infer that something in the construction of the dam may be interfering with the locals' biology. It is a well-known fact that when pollutants enter rivers, lakes, and streams, locals often experience lowered sperm counts, among other issues. Plastics containing estrogens that leach into water can effectively render fish and amphibians sterile. When medicine men say the god is departing, we may assume that a wealth of problems will result. Sacredness and the balance of a natural order often go hand-in-hand, especially when dealing with issues of birth and fertility.

Asia

In Asia, where rice has been the staple of life since civilization began there, it is no wonder that rice and fertility are inexorably intertwined. A trip through the winding emerald green rice terraces of Bali uncovers myriad devotional images of the loving rice goddess, Dewi Sri. During special festivals, the holy rice is attached to the forehead, much in the same way that ashes are applied to the heads of Christians during Lent.

In Thailand, the spirit of the rice is called Mae Posop, or "Rice Mother." When rice plants begin to seed, the Thai people say that the rice "becomes pregnant." The farmer offers bananas, fruits, and sugarcane for her morning sickness. He also brings toilet powder, a comb, and perfume to beautify one of the rice plants symbolically, praying to the spirit of the rice mother as he performs the ritual ablutions. Even after rice is farmed and cooked, the Goddess Mother must be invoked. If you want to tell your host that the rice is overcooked or underdone, you must first beg the Rice Mother's pardon. You must do the same if you drop food or discard left-over rice.

In Japanese Shinto belief, rice is considered a *kami*, or minor god, and is represented as both male and female or androgynous. Inari is the spirit of fertility and is sometimes shown as a fox. According to a 1985 survey by the National Association of Shinto Shrines, 32,000 shrines—more than one-third of Shinto shrines in Japan—are dedicated to Inari, the spirit of fecundity. Even in modern-day Japan, the festivals associated with this deity are hugely popular and have even grown in size. Along with bringing babies to families, Inari also brings success and other aspects of bounty. It follows that in Japan the words for "breakfast," "lunch," and "dinner" are "morning," "afternoon," and "evening rice."

Ireland: Holy Wells and Sacred Flames

Ireland has long been perceived as home to lingering folk beliefs long gone from most modern countries. This is partly true but changing quickly. As the European Union homogenizes member countries and what is called the Celtic Tiger business boom transforms the countryside into a mass of second homes and corporate headquarters, many of the folkways we associate with Ireland—fairies and leprechauns—have disappeared.

Some of Ireland's strongest folk beliefs—the ones that are hard to root out, even with technology and an improved economy—are the fertility rituals connected with the ancient Celtic goddess Brighid. Brighid (who was later morphed into a Catholic saint called St. Bridget) is associated with poetry, fertility, cows, and sacred flames, such as the one maintained by nineteen nuns at her sanctuary in County Kildare.

Her sacred flame at Kildare was said to have been surrounded by a hedge, which no man could cross. Men who attempted to cross the hedge were said to have been cursed to go insane, die, and/or to have had their "lower leg" wither. Brighid was also connected to holy wells, at Kildare and many other sites in the Celtic lands. Well dressing—the tying of rags to the trees next to healing wells—and other methods of petitioning or honoring Brighid for fertility and other boons is a practice still very much alive in Ireland. "Dressing" or laying flowers at a holy well is still a living practice in Ireland and one that is originally connected with fertility cults. Women also tie rags to sacred trees near the holy well, wishing for healthy babies. All over Ireland, you can still find sacred wells and when you find them, the trees nearby will inevitably be festooned with wishing rags—many of them placed with the hope of a newborn child.

Today, the site of Brighid's original flame is a cathedral churchyard. The nuns who care for the cathedral and the site keep a small prayer house where they tend the light of a modern version of the eternal flame.

Another connection all Irish women had to the goddess of fire and fertility was the tending of a similar fire in the home. This was considered a ritual that only women should perform, and special prayers were said that bound the sayer to the Celtic fertility rituals of ancient times. Women would stir the embers of the smoking peat in the fireplace and chant over the dying light every evening, praying to protect their homes and their children. Here is an example of one such prayer:

The sacred Three
To save,
To shield,
To surround
The hearth,
The house,
The household,
This eve,
This night,
Oh! this eve,
This night,
And every night,
Each single night.
      Amen.[4]

Latin America: The Leche Shrine

In St. Augustine, Florida, at the Mission of Nombre de Dios, the oldest Catholic church in the United States, the worship of Maria Lactans, or Mary as nursing mother, continues uninterrupted as it has in Europe for centuries.

The history of the devotion to the mother of Jesus as Our Lady of La Leche may have roots in a fourth-century grotto in Bethlehem. To this day the Franciscan community maintains a shrine there called the Milk Grotto. Its centerpiece is an image of the Blessed Virgin nursing the infant Jesus. Many believe that the crusaders brought the devotion to Mary as a nursing mother to Spain in the Middle Ages.

During the reign of Phillip III in Spain, word spread of a nobleman's pregnant wife who was expected to die during childbirth but was spared as a result of the intercession of Nuestra Senora de la Leche y Buen Parto (Our Lady of the Milk and Happy Delivery). The statue of this saint, in possession of the nobleman, soon found a place in the imaginations of many throughout Spain.

By the early 1600s, the devotion, under the title of Nuestra Senora de la Leche y Buen Parto, had become a part of the spiritual life of the Spanish settlers and the converted native peoples in St. Augustine. It was on these same mission grounds that the Spanish built the first Marian shrine in the land, and devotion to it continues to this day.

Thousands of visitors and pilgrims make their way to the shrine every year. Many ask for the blessings of motherhood, praying for the intercession of Our Lady of La Leche that God will grant them a safe and happy delivery and healthy children. Many write requesting remembrances in masses and prayers not only for motherhood but for petitions of all kinds. Other sites devoted to the image of Mary as nursing mother exist around the country, but the church at St. Augustine is the oldest and has been most closely associated with "miracles," such as infertile couples getting pregnant.

> PRAYER TO OUR LADY OF LA LECHE, LOVELY LADY OF LA LECHE, most loving Mother of the Child Jesus, and my mother, listen to my humble prayer. Your motherly heart knows my every wish, my every need. To you only, his spotless Virgin Mother, has your Divine Son given to understand the sentiments which fill my soul. Yours was the sacred privilege of being the Mother of the Savior. Intercede with him now, my loving mother, that, in accordance with his will, I may become the mother of other children of our heavenly Father.[5]

Ixchel, Fertility, and the Rain Forest

In the Mayan world, the goddess of fertility was called Ixchel, the snake goddess of water and the moon, of childbirth, and of weaving. She was married to the earth god Voltan but fell in love with the moon god Itzamna, considered the founder of the Mayans because he taught them how to read, write, and grow corn. When Ixchel became his consort, she gave birth to four powerful sons known as the Bacabs, who continue to hold up the sky in each of the four directions. Sometimes called Lady Rainbow, Ixchel controls the tides and all water on earth. She is also the first lady of medicine and brings healing to humans through plants, water, and other natural remedies. Often portrayed as a wise crone, she is seen wearing a skirt decorated with crossbones and a crown of serpents while carrying a jug of water. The crossbones are a symbol of her role as the giver of new life and keeper of dead souls. The serpents represent her wisdom and power to rejuvenate. The water jug alludes to her dual role as both a benign and destructive deity. Although she gives humankind the continual gift of water—the most essential element of life—according to Mayan myth, Ixchel also sent floods to cleanse the earth of wicked men who had stopped thanking the gods. She is said to give special protection to those making the sacred pilgrimage to her sites in Cozumel and Isla Mujeres.

Belize is a small Central American country formerly known as British Honduras with nearly two-thirds of its tropical rain forests intact. It is considered to be the heartland of the ancient Mayan civilization. It is in Belize that Dr. Rosita Arvigo, an herbalist and researcher, has named a foundation after Ixchel. The Ix Chel Tropical Rainforest Foundation was created after Arvigo's work with a local shaman/healer revealed to her the myriad ways in which local herbs and other natural methods were used in traditional healing. Arvigo apprenticed with a local shaman/healer named Don Elijio Panti and wrote a book about her experiences, *Satsun*. A large part of her work with Don Elijio was in what she called "Mayan Abdominal Massage." This technique, which she now teaches as the "Arvigo Technique," uses traditional movements to massage the abdomen. Some of the results Arvigo claims are healthier pregnancies and enhanced fertility. Dr. Arvigo's work is a fascinating example of how ancient rites and fertility traditions combine with science and conservation. The original fertility myths of Ixchel are experiencing a transformative renaissance in the modern world—truly a fusion of myth, magic, and medicine.

Aboriginal Beliefs about Birth: Spirit Babies

In Australian aboriginal belief, birth is a powerful time when unseen spirits find a way into the world and choose to be born. In traditional aboriginal belief, if a mother goes to a sacred space filled with spirit such as Uluru (formerly Ayers Rock), she can "invite" spirit into her in the form of a child. It is thus understood that the spirit inherent in a place where conception took place may have bearing on the nature of a child. So if you find your child is conceived at sea and ultimately has a deep love for the ocean, the aboriginal belief would say that ocean spirits were responsible for his or her conception. Some aboriginal beliefs also hold that the umbilical cord should be planted beneath a sacred tree and that a portion of the cord is wound like a necklace around the baby's neck. Another intriguing aspect of aboriginal childbirth belief is the concept that animal spirits may play a part in the child's conception. Mothers "consider their role in childbirth as that of an agent or temporary transit for a being with its own spiritual pre-existence."[6] Consequently, if a child is aborted or miscarries, they believe that spirit will try to be born again—either with the same mother or in a different place.

The Philippines—The Obando Dances

In the Philippines, the Obando Dances are a modern-day Filipino fertility ritual. Every year during the month of May, the men, women, and children of Obando, Bulacan, wear traditional dance costumes and dance on the streets followed by the images of their patron saints San Pascual Baylon (St. Paschal), Santa Clara (St. Clare), and Nuestra Señora de Salambao (Our Lady of Salambao), while singing the song "Santa Clara Pinung-Pino."

Among the fiesta participants in the fertility dance are outsiders from other towns in the Philippines, most of whom are asking the patron saints for a son or a daughter, a husband or a wife, or good fortune. They all dance on the streets in order for the spirit of life to enter into the wombs of women.

The feast usually starts on the morning of May 17, with a mass conducted by the current parish priest. Then begins the procession of the three saints, followed by the dancing of the devotees and the musical band. This continues for the duration of the festival, with the image of the particular patron saint of the day leading the procession.

The ancient Filipinos held a ritual known as the Kasilonawan headed by a *katalonan*, or high priestess. The ritual, usually held at the home of a *datu* or *barangay* chieftain, lasted for about nine days and usually involved drinking, singing, and dancing. The ritual became important to early Filipinos because they valued fertility, which could also mean wealth or abundance of every individual. A barren woman was once considered a member of the lowest class in Filipino society and suffered stigma and mockery. Because of this, it became important to perform the fertility rites so that the women could become productive. The god known as Linga, a force of nature, became the center of the Kasilonawan ritual.

The community would usually congregate to perform these rituals in a clearing of some kind in the middle of a dense forest with some sort of earth-oriented and artistic phallic symbol displayed in the center of the clearing. The lights of strategically placed ritualistic fires would shine on this structure, and it was thought that the sun, giver of all life embodied in the fires, was giving its blessing of fertility to all who participated in the rituals.

When the Franciscan missionaries came to the Philippines, they built churches to propagate Christianity and introduced Catholic saints. In Obando, Bulacan, the Spanish Franciscans introduced a trio of saints: St. Claire, St. Pascual, and Our Lady of Salambao in order to replace the traditional pagan gods.

The current images at the altar of Obando Church are replicas, sculpted with the financial assistance of the people of Obando. The originals were destroyed during World War II.

The Obando is an example of a tribe fusing ancient animistic fertility rites with newer Catholic traditions brought to the Philippines by the Spanish. They are a vibrant illustration of the ways in which ancient rites of passage are still relevant to in modern-day people's lives.

Rites of Passage in Everyday Life

As we've seen, global traditions of childbirth and fertility have not entirely been abandoned by people in favor of modern medicine. In most cases where such traditions still exist, they do so in tandem with modern medicine, something that I am all in favor of.

If your own culture's myths have an emotional resonance for you, there is no reason to completely turn your back on them as "superstition" or "heathen" beliefs. Psychologist Carl Jung and writer/philosopher Joseph Campbell have both popularized a new way to look at myths: as stories that tell emotional truths about us as people. As Campbell himself said, "Every religion is true one way or another. It is true when understood metaphorically. But when it gets stuck in its own metaphors, interpreting them as facts, then you are in trouble."[7]

Other helpful aspects of traditional healing and beliefs in childbirth and fertility include balance, respect for the environment, and continuity with the ways of nature and the experiences of our ancestors.

I would encourage you to explore the myth-conceptions, stories, and legends of childbirth that are associated with your own heritage and culture. You can listen to the stories, songs, and poems of your foremothers and fathers and bring the positive aspects of them into the story of your own pregnancy. Myths and legends are no substitute for good, modern medical care, but their existence makes the experience richer and deeper. Knowing the lore of the people you come from binds you and your child to them in a way that can only enhance your pregnancy and your experience of childbirth. And it gives you great bedtime stories to tell your children and your children's children.

Global Deities of Fertility and Childbirth

Egyptian

Tawret. The hippopotamus "midwife" goddess who helps pregnant women in childbirth

Isis. Mother goddess seen in statues with baby Horus on her knee

Hathor/Sekmet. Fertility goddess and helper of pregnant women

Bes. Dwarf god who keeps newborn children from crying with his antics

Roman

The Romans had a panoply of gods and goddesses who attended the newborn. Here are some of the most interesting ones:

Opigena. Aids in childbirth

Natio. Aids in childbirth (from the root word also seen in *natal*)

Vaticanus. God who helps stop crying newborns

Educa. Procures food for the baby

Rumina. Goddess of breastfeeding

Potina. Brings baby medicine

Vitummus. Gives life to fetus

Sentinus. Gives sensation to fetus

Cunina. Guardian of the cradle

Ossipage. Hardens the bones of the infant

Statulinus. Helps newborns to walk

Lucina. Aids mother in labor

Partula. Presides over delivery

Carmentis. Predicts future of newborn (like the good fairy in the story of Sleeping Beauty)

Levana. Protects the child when it is lifted up and sees that the father accepts the child (in Roman tradition, a father had to lift his infant in his arms to declare it as truly his)

Locutius. Taught infants to speak (not just the name of Captain Picard as a "Borg" in the film *Star Trek: The Next Generation*)

Greek

Artemis/Diana. Virgin goddess of the moon, protectress of all animals (and humans) when bearing young. She is sometimes seen as a multibreasted woman with enough milk to feed all of humanity, and goddess of love and all things connected with it, including fertility.

Demeter. The goddess of single mothers. She lost her daughter Persephone to the god of the dead and was permitted to be with her daughter for only half of the year (spring). When Persephone had to go back to Hades, Demeter mourned, and the season turned to winter.

Juno. Mother of the gods (with Zeus) and protectress of married women and mothers. Maybe her stories explain why the name Juno was chosen for the recent film about a single teen mother.

African (including diaspora gods in United States, Brazil, Cuba)

Yemanya. Fishtail goddess of the ocean and fertility, maybe one reason African Americans say to dream of a fish is to predict a child being born.

Erzulie Frida. Goddess of love, sex, and fertility in Yoruba/Santeria/*voudon*. She is prayed to for all things connected with love.

Oshun. Goddess of rivers and fertility

Shango. Twin god, fertility icon, and bringer of thunder

Asian

India

> **Ganesha.** Opener of the way, breaker of obstacles (to childbirth)
> **Sarasvati.** The "flowing" goddess of rivers and also fertility
> **Krishna and Radha.** Divine couple who are constantly embracing and making love
> **Shiva.** Medicine and fertility, his penis is worshipped as the "lingam"

China

> **Chang-O.** Goddess of the moon and fertility
> **Kwan Yin.** Goddess of mercy

Japan

> **Kannon.** Goddess of mercy, love, and fertility

Central America

> **Ixchel.** Mayan goddess of medicine and miracles, also fertility
> **Chac.** Mayan fertility rain god

Europe

> **Freya.** Nordic goddess of cats, love, and fertility.
> **Brighid.** Celtic/Irish goddess of the hearth, home, and fertility
> **St. Catherine of Sweden.** Patron saint of miscarriage prevention
> **St. Gerard Majella.** Patron saint of pregnancy and expectant mothers
> **St. Raymund Nonnatus.** Patron saint of midwives

Notes

1. Kathleen A. Costigan, Heather L. Sipsma, and Janet A. DiPietro, "Pregnancy Folklore Revisited: The Case of Heartburn and Hair," *Birth* 33, no. 4 (2006): 311.

2. BBC News, September 8, 2008.

3. Interview by journalist Gretchen Kelly with local medicine man.

4. http://www.sacred-texts.com/neu/celt/cg1/index.htm (accessed April 22, 2009).

5. http://www.missionandshrine.org/la_leche.htm (accessed April 22, 2009).

6. Robert Lawlor, *Voices of the First Day* (Rochester, VT: Inner Traditions, 1991).

7. http://www.brainyquote.com/quotes/quotes/j/josephcamp139169.html (accessed April 26, 2009).

Section Six

The Seven Habits to a Highly Enjoyable Pregnancy

Chapter Thirteen

The Seven Habits to a Highly Enjoyable Pregnancy

I n our Western culture and cultures throughout the world, the number seven has spiritual, emotional, and literal significance. A recent search on Amazon.com brought up 410,212 items with the number seven in the product title. Many books with the number seven in the title have gone on to become best sellers. Before we learn the seven habits to a highly enjoyable pregnancy, let's take a brief detour into the number seven itself.

First and foremost, we would like to bring the reader's attention to the Seven Deadly Sins: Pride, Envy, Gluttony, Lust, Anger, Greed, and Sloth. Many women reading this book will recognize that they may have progressed through some of these Seven Deadly Sins through the short cycle of their pregnancy—possibly all in one day. The seven habits to a highly enjoyable pregnancy may not directly invoke the Seven Deadly Sins, but they will indirectly summon the power of your pregnancy to combat potential obstacles. It is our hope that through the seven habits your pregnancy will be easier and more enjoyable. Here are the Seven Deadly Sins and how they pertain to pregnant women:

- **Pride.** "Inordinate self-love is the cause of every sin... the root of pride is found to consist in man not being, in some way, subject to God and his rule" ST 1:77 (Summa Theologica).*

   Pride has a negative connotation in our society, but pride in one-self can be a good thing. As a pregnant woman, if you are able to contemplate on the upcoming joys of a new baby or the fascinating changes occurring in your body, this could be a prideful, and powerful, feeling of self-actualization.

- **Envy.** Here is an example of how envy affected one of our pregnant patients.

   > J. A., a beautiful twenty-four-year-old woman pregnant at about thirty weeks, came to the office for a routine obstetrical visit. She started her pregnancy at about 125 pounds and was currently 140 pounds, with the baby measuring appropriately; basically a healthy pregnancy and patient. She asked if she was gaining enough weight. When asked why she was worried about her weight gain, she said that some of her friends and coworkers were telling her that she was too small and needed to gain weight for her baby. This can happen to smaller women who might be the object of envy of some of their more overweight family and friends. There is an assumption that the smaller pregnant woman should be gaining weight, and envy ensues when friends see that she can still be happy, healthy, and small. This can cause significant anxiety in patients because they feel as though they are not eating enough and are potentially harming their babies. Healthy weight gain during a pregnancy is twenty-five to thirty-five pounds throughout the forty-week pregnancy. In some instances, women will lose weight if they are overweight at the beginning of the pregnancy. As physicians we measure the abdomen at every visit to confirm that the baby is growing appropriately. In many instances, weight gain of the mother does not reflect weight gain of the baby. Pregnant women should concern themselves only with their own health and the health of their baby—not what their envious friends say.

---

*The Summa Theologica was written by Catholic saint Francis of Assisi.

- **Gluttony.** Gluttony is an inordinate desire to consume more than one requires. There are obviously gluttonous behaviors that do not relate to eating, but excessive food and drink in pregnancy is a hot topic. The basic premise of "all things in moderation" is a good philosophy to live by. Some things should be avoided during pregnancy, like alcohol and drugs, but what about diet drinks, juices, caffeine, high-fat foods? One cup of coffee, a glass of juice, or a hamburger is not going to throw your pregnancy into a tailspin; some things in moderation help to keep you sane.

- **Lust.** For many, lust or sexual desire during pregnancy may decrease at certain points. In the first trimester, with its attendant nausea and vomiting, it may be difficult to feel like a sexual being. The third trimester, "the big bag of hurt," is rife with low-back pain, varicose veins, swelling of the ankles, vaginal discharge, and an overall feeling of discomfort; this also does not promote a healthy libido. The glorious second trimester, when nausea calms down and the hormones have finally stabilized, may be a time when women are at their sexual peak during pregnancy. This can change for women throughout the pregnancy and can vary from woman to woman.

- **Anger.** Who doesn't get angry? Mood and personality take on a different form as the pregnant woman moves further into the maternal archetype. As we all know, there are times when mothers are nurturing, caring, kind, and attentive. There are also times when the mother must be the disciplinarian or must punish the child. It is important to take note of mood swings during pregnancy. A flash of anger can simply be irritability, or it may be the presenting emotion for something more serious, like depression. We would recommend simple adjustments for mood swings, like getting plenty of sleep, regular low-impact physical activity, eating well, taking naps, trying yoga or meditation. If severe mood swings last longer than two weeks, we recommend that you speak to your physician or health-care provider.

- **Greed.** Like pride, greed tends to convey a negative feeling or behavior pattern in our culture. Maternal greed tends to manifest more as a desire to control the care of the infant. In other words, you might become greedy about your baby; this is the protecting mechanism called maternal instinct. There may also be a desire to join the ranks of the tribe of motherhood. Motherhood is the ultimate tribe that has one stringent requirement: a baby. Other tribelike qualities are a profound lack of sleep, a small loss of control (babies don't listen), and a deep sense of purpose.

• **Sloth.** Most pregnant women are tired, not slothful. Many pregnant women are on bed rest because of doctor's orders, not because they're lazy.

Besides the Seven Deadly Sins, there are the Seven Heavenly Virtues (Faith, Hope, Charity, Fortitude, Justice, Temperance, and Prudence), the Seven Contrary Virtues (Humility, Kindness, Abstinence, Chastity, Patience, Liberality, Diligence), the Seven Catholic Sacraments, the Seven Chakras,* and seven levels to the Tree of Life in Kabbalah.

As you can see, the significance of the number seven was not just invented by the self-help industry. The number seven actually has great importance in many religious and cultural traditions and as such can be viewed as a sort of guide. This guide can be applied to pregnancy, which we will show in this chapter.

When Shawn was in his residency at the University of Oklahoma, he taught a review course for third-year medical students on their ob-gyn rotation. The students would engage in a discussion about the multitude of topics they had learned and ask questions about their upcoming exam. Many of the students liked to discuss topics that seemed more prevalent in the lay press and magazine articles. In an effort to expand upon the power of myth and superstition, we would like to elaborate on the power of personal belief systems, family, community, friends, and expectations. All of these influences have been boiled down into seven formulated rules or habits that can help you have a highly enjoyable pregnancy.

1. Do not watch daytime talk shows or read women's health magazines.
2. Be nice but don't listen to Grandma.
3. Listen to the good birthing stories, but beware of the battle-hardened birth veterans.
4. Honor thy family; stay connected.

---

*The chakras are energy centers in the body and an important part of Eastern Indian mystical traditions. The chakras are arranged on the body from head to foot, and each one influences a certain aspect of the individual's psychospiritual life.

5. Understand your voice; avoid the herd mentality.
6. You're expecting, so expect nothing.
7. Ask questions: Explore, educate, enjoy.

1. Do Not Watch Daytime Talk Shows or Read Women's Health Magazines

The following quote comes from an interview with actress Julia Roberts on the *Oprah Winfrey* show.[1] Ms. Roberts had just admitted to being nervous about the fact that she was soon to be a parent. "What if I didn't know that I wasn't supposed to feed the babies honey in their first year of life—because of bacteria. What if I did not know that I wasn't supposed to eat peanuts?"

These two statements made by Julia Roberts in front of millions of viewers (I am assuming thousands of whom are pregnant) provoked fear in some of the pregnant patients we saw in our office.

There is definitely concern with giving babies raw honey early in life, mainly because raw organic honey has not gone through a pasteurization process, and so there is a risk of botulism. Concern arose when it was found that raw organic honey may contain spores that, under the right circumstances, contain a rare deadly disease discovered in 1976 called infantile botulism. Infantile botulism is spread by spores, not by preformed botulism toxin. If you give your infant honey in her early years, pasteurized products will more than likely be free of these spores due to the heating of the pasteurization process. Also worth remembering, many parents give their infants honey because they believe it is better than sugar, but sweet is sweet, and honey is just another form of a simple sugar.

The second statement made by Ms. Roberts concerns not eating peanuts while pregnant. Even as we write this, we still have patients who ask this question, although they are unsure where they heard it. There is open debate that women who eat peanuts during pregnancy can have children who develop peanut allergies. If you are a purist, then you may wish to avoid peanuts altogether, since data on children with peanut allergies are inconclusive. There are other nuts that make a healthy snack and do not carry the potential allergens (cashews and walnuts), but they might be processed in a factory that also uses peanuts and thus might convey the allergen.

We believe that Ms. Roberts was unknowingly making reference to an obscure toxin called aflatoxin, which is produced by fungus on some peanuts. A study done in 1966 showed that pregnant rats exposed to aflatoxin had no fetal or placental effects other than a slightly decreased birth weight.[2]

Aflatoxin is a naturally occurring toxin produced by a mold and can occur also on corn. We have yet to have anyone ask about the safety of corn in her diet when pregnant. In the United States, federal and state inspections, as well as proper storage and transportation, reduce the risk of aflatoxin in the human food supply. Basically, the issues with aflatoxin exposure from peanuts is more of a third world issue. It is indeed a real concern and has been described as a carcinogen if consumed in large quantities. Personally, we feel that peanuts are a good source of protein and if eaten in a responsible manner are a healthy addition to a pregnant woman's diet. If you make radical changes to your diet after becoming pregnant, you may wind up bloated, undernourished, and miserable until your body adjusts to your new regimen.

We titled this section with our tongues firmly in our cheeks, partly because our society barrages us on a daily basis with information from the Internet, cell phones, television, and other forms of marketing. Many of the headlines and recommendations concerning health are made in a frightening or confusing way. We recommend the habit of avoiding women's magazines and daytime talk shows because these mediums tend to send shockwaves through the pregnant community. We still get questions about peanuts three years after this interview between Oprah and Julia Roberts; there are partial truths and real concerns. Most, if not all, pregnant women are concerned with the well-being of their baby and want answers to address that concern. What one needs to discover early in pregnancy is that physicians, midwives, doulas, and other women's health experts are excellent sources of information. We would also recommend that when you are presented with information that seems threatening or questionable, you ask yourself a few questions:

- Could this possibly be a familial or cultural superstition?
- Have I asked my healthcare provider about this?
- Have I heard this information before, and if so, what are the sources?

The main point to recommending that you avoid women's magazines and daytime talk shows is to reconnect you with the information you get from your body. By focusing your attention on those things outside of your body (such as the constant barrage of white noise and twenty-four-hour news channels), you are dissociating from your own antenna. We hear so many women make the simple statement that they feel their baby move more when they take the time to lie down. When you are busy and engaged in repetitive behaviors of the daily chores and work, you are not mindful of the baby inside of you. The joy of pregnancy is, quite simply, being pregnant. Just like you can become disconnected with your own pregnancy, women have fallen prey to medicine's disconnect. Are mind and body separate or the same? This is the question that cannot be answered by simple science or religion.

In order to set a firm foundation for your pregnancy, you should consider daily practices that connect mind and body; not just your own mind-body connection but that with the baby developing within you. When you have those quiet times with your unborn baby, listen to your own breath and realize that same oxygen is going to your baby; the exhaling breath is not only eliminating your carbon dioxide but also that of your baby. Be mindful of the food you are eating and realize that as it is digested, it is going directly to your baby to help nourish him or her. Reacting with fear to information on the news and in magazines can stem from monetary issues, housing and employment changes, and relationships. Fear can turn into anxiety and can contribute to a host of problems, from insomnia and fatigue to high blood pressure.

Take a break from the television and reconnect with your body by experiencing a prenatal massage, walking in nature, meditating, or doing yoga. Take care of yourself inside and out.

2. Be Nice, but Don't Listen to Grandma

Shawn grew up in a Catholic American family in the Berkshires of Massachusetts. On his mother's side, the family was governed by the matriarch, his grandmother; his grandfather made special appearances on the holidays. He and his two cousins would meet at their grandmother's house, like tribal initiates, every Tuesday at around 6:00 p.m. for dinner. The dinner would always take the form of hamburgers, homemade French fries, and soda. The hamburgers were of the leanest beef and were perfectly pressed into circles long before Tupperware invented the patty maker; Grandma also cut the fries by hand. There was never a Tuesday that this gathering did not take place with all participants at the same table in their designated seats. The point of this story is twofold: to show the power of ritual and to emphasize the power of the matriarch. Shawn's Tuesday dinner ritual was always headed by his grandmother; in many families, the head matriarch is the grandmother. The matriarch can be like the benevolent queen and rule with grace, or she can be dictatorial and risk her people rising and revolting. In many cases, the role of grandmother is its own archetype and wields a mighty power, often with an iron fist, if not clothed in a matronly garb of loose-fitting housedresses and hairnets. Shawn's grandmother is only five foot one, but people feared, respected, and loved her. It has been noted that grandmothers contribute to many myths surrounding pregnancy, and we have discovered that even a medical degree pales in comparison to the RG (Reigning Grandmother) degree. To illustrate the power of the grandmother and her relationship to pregnancy, we would like to share the following experience:

B. R. was a nineteen-year-old Hispanic female who was diagnosed with a breech baby (baby's feet were presenting instead of the head). The patient's grandmother had instructed her granddaughter that the reason the baby was in the breech position was because the patient had moved around too much in her pregnancy (obviously jostling the baby into this position). These accusations made B. R. blame herself for the fact that the baby was in this position. In cases where the baby is breech, most physicians will offer the patient the chance to undergo a procedure called an external version, or to simply schedule a cesarean section. B. R. had opted for the external version, in which we try to turn the baby by manipulating the pregnant abdomen. The success rate of this procedure is around 50 percent, and B. R. had a successful procedure. With her baby now turned to a head-down position, B. R.'s grandmother instructed her to "not move around so much." When the patient was brought to labor and delivery in active labor, she was in excruciating pain and requesting an epidural. The nurse told me that the patient wanted an epidural but she was desperately afraid of the side effects. I had remembered talking with the patient about the epidural during her pregnancy and was surprised to hear this, as she had not stated any concerns with the procedure prior to this point.

I arrived at the patient's room and was privy to the scene of a queen and her court. The patient was on the birthing bed in horrible pain with her two sisters at either side, holding her legs in a flexed position. B. R.'s mother (the grandmother-to-be) was standing approximately three feet to the patient's left side, and the patient's grandmother was sitting in a chair in the corner of the room, her arms folded across her chest in a dominant gesture. In the ceremonial tradition, I put on my gown and took my seat as the delivering physician (knowing I was not the one in control). My patient had the look on her face that she was between worlds. I was instructing her on how to focus and push through the pain; she wouldn't push. Her sisters spoke softly to her and told her that it was time for the baby to come out and her little one needed her to push; she still would not push. From the corner of the room, the grandmother stated, "It is normal to feel pain, mija. It is time to have the baby." On the next contraction, B. R. pushed with all her energy and gave birth to a healthy baby girl, at which point the grandmother walked over to the sisters and told them to talk to their new niece. I realized at that time that the medical degree was nothing compared to the power of a grandmother and matriarch.

The case above is descriptive of the power of family dynamics in pregnancy. Family dynamics in pregnancy and labor and delivery are concerned with sexuality, sensuality, fertility, creative life energy, and the power of our personal relationships. In the case of pregnancy and the matriarchal family dynamic, there is a dominant female figure dictating the course of action for the protection of the laboring patient under her control.

Women with a strong maternal bond have a connection to the mothers in their past. Myths revolving around the birthing process can be helpful to healthcare providers by aiding them in birthing plans and helping them interact with the family and patient during the delivery process. We do not make light of the fact that myths passed down through grandmothers may hold special significance to a patient and her culture, and at times, these myths can help with such things as pain control and support after the delivery. These myths may help new mothers bond with their maternal ancestors and bring forth belief structures that will help in the postpartum care of the child. A strong female presence in the delivery room is essential on many levels.

There can, however, be problems when this governing maternal figure is at odds with the patient. Those patients with distant relationships to their mothers or grandmothers, and thus their maternal ancestry, may find it difficult to understand why their grandmother is telling them not to get an epidural. This could cause stress and anxiety in the delivery room.

We have found that one of the best ways to make the most of the dominant female figure in the delivery room is to try to involve her in the care of her loved one; that is why we jokingly state that you should be respectful and listen to your grandmother, but sometimes you have to make your own decisions. The labor and delivery experience is a creative process for the mother and family, and any strain in this area can dampen the joy of the birth. If there is anxiety in the room, the laboring patient may be more focused on her pain and fear.

Unfortunately, many teenagers today become pregnant, an act that will obviously challenge the family structure. The young mother may feel that she has violated a familial and cultural taboo by becoming sexual at a young age, and the pregnancy can be a reminder to her of that betrayal to her family structure. Many times the matriarch or ruling female figure may also have feelings of guilt because she may feel she was not there to educate her daughter or granddaughter, but through the pregnancy and delivery process she can definitely dictate the course of action.

Why then would a grandmother or maternal figure tell a pregnant mother not to get an epidural because it could paralyze or injure her? We have seen in a previous chapter that an epidural has a very small risk profile, but there are risks and side effects. There are many reasons a matriarchal figure might warn against an epidural, some of which are cultural, mythical, and personal. I have heard grandmothers say, "They didn't have epidurals when I had kids...I just dealt with the pain" to which patients responded, "Yeah, but they didn't have television back then and you watch it now." This is not an argument any physician likes to get involved in.

It may be that some matriarchs regard the labor and delivery process as anything but a pleasurable experience; that is why they call it "labor." On this view, the way into the tribe of motherhood is to become a card-carrying member of the "pain club." This "easy way out" of the labor process with epidurals can be perceived by the elder women in a family as insufficient for acceptance into the tribe of motherhood. Some patients feel that if they do not experience the pain of labor, their bonding with the infant won't be as strong. However, we often see women who opt out of an epidural screaming with pain throughout their labor, and when the moment of delivery occurs, they are so exhausted they do not want the baby with them. On the other hand, we see women in labor who, thanks to an epidural, are able to push their baby out while looking into a mirror. If pain was really an inherent part of the birthing process, then what does this say about the woman who undergoes a cesarean section? There is definitely an argument that the cesarean section rate is too high and that the surgical process can interfere with proper bonding.

We would recommend listening to the elder females because they have years of experience in motherhood and they can be helpful getting you through the labor process. Take from them their nuggets of information and tuck them away for future use. We firmly believe in the fact that every woman has a different experience and that women need to listen to their own inner voice when deciding what is right for them. People around you may try to influence your decision based on their own personal experiences, but by listening to your instincts, you will know your path when the time comes.

Gaining control during the birthing process is a means to decrease pain and increase satisfaction. Empowerment can often be discovered through personal inner strength. In an effort to empower our patients in the birthing process, we ask them to engage in artistic endeavors to explore the beauty around them. Writing, painting, journaling, and music are such endeavors, and they can open you up to your surroundings and also help you focus your attention on your baby. There is evidence to show that your unborn baby can benefit from external musical stimulation. A 1975 study showed that Brahm's "Lullaby" played six times a day for five minutes in a nursery of premature babies resulted in a faster weight gain than other ambient sounds.[3] Researchers in Belfast also demonstrated that fetal audition can be demonstrated at sixteen weeks' gestation.[4]

So how do you know when the matriarch is starting to invade your pregnancy? Take a look at the checklist below:

- Are you receiving information that is going against plans or goals you originally wanted to accomplish? Is this information coming from the older women in your family?
- Is this information causing a strain in your relationship?
- Do you feel that there are any physical drives that are controlling you? Do you feel like you are trying to control things in your life? Obvi-

ously, control can be completely normal, and we are making reference to things that are making you overly possessive or controlling.

In those times when you feel like your self-control is being taken away from you by family members and friends, you might try things like mindful meditation or simply lying down for an hour and feeling your baby's movements, sensing how your pregnant body feels from head to toe, and being thankful for the decisions you have made so far.

How do you deal with controlling maternal figures in your family who are trying to decide for you how your pregnancy will proceed? Part of the healing process is a movement toward personal liberation, which in turn is a move toward personal independence and rebirth. As you try to connect with your own familial tribe, you are also attempting to establish yourself as an expert of your body. The role of the family should be one of support and education, but when there is also collective guilt, we recommend that you step back and reassess your desires. We have devised a Pregnant Woman's Bill of Rights to help you during your pregnancy.

Pregnant Woman's Bill of Rights

1. The pregnant woman is emotional. While there may be emotions that have surfaced since the beginning of the pregnancy, this in no way condemns her to nine months of guilt. She will have emotions ranging from sadness to anger, yet these are part of the natural process of becoming a mother.
2. As emotions ebb and flow, the pregnant woman can choose to release them or look to her social network for support.
3. The pregnant woman understands that there will be times when emotions can rage on their own and times she may feel the need for support.
4. The pregnant woman retains her sexuality. Her sexuality may require a balance and personal nurturing. The pregnant state is not a state of being "broken" but of being different. The pregnant woman retains the right to remain an individual. While she understands that she has a baby under her care, she is not the baby, and the baby is not her. She deserves respect for her individuality.
5. The pregnant woman has a right to her own birthing plan.

3. Listen to the Good Birthing Stories, but Beware of the Battle-Hardened Birth Veterans

Even physicians have to admit that there are times when we simply do not have good answers to some of these questions—most of which come from a friend or family member of the patient. We have often felt that there should be a Trivial Pursuit game for pregnancy. Undoubtedly, some women would be wizards at this game because of their own trials and tribulations during their pregnant journeys. They have survived the rigors of a difficult pregnancy and have lived to tell their tale. It seems that there is a previously unknown society of women elders who have organized and developed a knowledge of pregnancy based on their collective stories. This society has ranks within itself and accepts new women based on their stories. We call these women Knights of the Belly. These Knights of the Belly are the protectors of the meek and weary. They are ever-ready to defend their sisters with their swords of truth. The problem with the Knights is that they are difficult to defeat and practically invincible when they are protecting a pregnant damsel in distress. We call this group the Knights of the Belly to emphasize the fact that these women are the battle-hardened pregnancy veterans; the women who have been through pregnancy, delivery, and who have no problem telling everyone within earshot the story of their travails. Any postpartum woman can be knighted into this special group, but those with a particularly dramatic pregnancy history rise higher in the ranks. We definitely do not mean to make light of these women who have indeed gone through a difficult pregnancy or labor. Rather, we are referencing those women who had a typical pregnancy with a good outcome but who focused on one or two particular points and dramatized them, similar to the fisherman who tells the tale of the one that got away. Here is an example of an encounter with one of the Knights of the Belly:

> It was a cold December night in the little town of Lawton, Oklahoma. There had been an ice storm, which is characteristic of Oklahoma winters, and the military base had shut down, making it difficult to leave or enter. Since the weather was particularly bad and I could not leave for the evening, I hunkered down in my office with a good book, hoping for a quiet night. I had barely made it through the inside cover of the book when my pager went off. The labor and delivery nurses described the

story of a twenty-two-year-old first-time mother who had come in after her bag of water had broken. The nurses had confirmed that indeed her bag of water was ruptured, but that the patient was denying any sort of IV, Pitocin, or other "invasive" hospital procedures. I remembered this woman's name but did not remember her telling me any of this during her antepartum care, and actually I remembered that she had told me she was definitely getting an epidural. I walked down to labor and delivery and found my patient in mild to moderate discomfort with a pained look on her face. In the corner of the room was a shadowed figure whom I will call Leslie. I did not know this at the time, but Leslie was a newly inducted Knight of the Belly; because of her knighthood, I feel like we should call her Leslie the Painful because she was there to make sure that the patient received no pain medication or any other intervention.

I asked my patient why she was refusing the pain medication and IV when she had not mentioned an aversion to pain control during our prior visits. She told me that the IV was okay, but that she did not want Pitocin because that would make her contractions stronger, and stronger contractions meant more painful labor. I agreed that if we had to give her Pitocin because of inadequate labor then indeed her contractions would increase and this could cause pain, but only the normal labor pains. With this information, my patient glanced over at Leslie the Painful, her support, then looked back over to me and said, "We are going natural." It was then that I realized that Leslie was a Knight of the Belly and that she had ridden in on her white minivan, with her helmet (a Yankees ball cap), and she was going to give me a rundown of the horrors of her pregnancy.

In a phrase, It was on.

Leslie stood complacently at the patient's side and began describing the travails of her own pregnancy.

"I had an epidural with my last child and ended up with a cesarean section," she said. I told her I sympathized with her and that sometimes things don't always turn out the way the patients expect them to in their birthing plans. I also told her that she might have ended up with a cesarean section even if she did not have the epidural. She sensed my challenge, but being a pure Knight of the Belly she was ready and brought forth her bevy of weapons. She pummeled me with her history, "Not only did I have a cesarean section, I was in the hospital for seven days with an infection, had a wound separation, and because of this my baby did not breastfeed well and had to go the bottle. I am still having numbness at my incision site." I immediately recognized that I would be unable to parry this entire melee and thus I backed down, lest I be emasculated right in front of my patient. You see, the Knight is full of purity and light, and during this confrontation I realized that this woman was not going to allow anything "bad" to happen to her friend. The epidural was a cult of its own, and the Knight was not going to let it take her friend.

Again, I expressed my sympathies and understanding to Leslie and then turned to ask my patient what she wanted to do; she again stated that she wished to proceed with natural childbirth. I want to go on record as saying that I feel natural childbirth is a wonderful process and that the women I have seen go through this process are some of the most impressive women I have met. In this particular case, however, I knew that my patient wanted to have pain control since we had talked about it just a week ago. I felt that she was not really speaking her mind for fear of upsetting her friend. Looking at my patient and almost expecting her to send me a message via Morse code eye blinks, I had an epiphany. Knights are noble and are willing to go to the ends of the earth for those under their protection. I had to send the Knight on a noble quest.

My patient's husband was in Bosnia on a peacekeeping mission and could not be present for the delivery of their first baby. I looked around the room and noticed that in the haste of leaving her house she had not brought anything of his to the room. I asked the patient if she had anything at the hospital that she could focus on that might help her get through the contractions, like a picture of her husband. She said through her bloodshot eyes, "Yes, I really could use a picture of Jim." I then turned to Leslie and asked if she would mind going back to the patient's house to get a picture of Jim to help her friend through the contractions. The Knight now had a holy grail and after smiling at the patient, she promptly left the room to begin her quest. With the bad weather and worse roads, she said it might take her an hour before she could get back. I don't think Leslie had even made it to her noble minivan before my patient asked the nurse to get her an epidural. I am not sure if Leslie realized that her friend had received an epidural when she returned, as she never said a word.

My patient had a wonderful delivery.

The point of this story is to emphasize that there are many women out there who have delivered babies and they all have stories. But these are not *your* stories. Women who have had uncomplicated, smooth deliveries with and without epidurals or medications are not knighted into the Bellyhood, and thus you usually do not hear from them; their stories, being fairly unremarkable, are not really worth telling. These women of easy deliveries may also fear that the Bellyhood would chastise them if they were to start talking about their easy deliveries, lest they convince all women that pregnancy is something to be taken lightly. The Knights of the Belly are very passionate and they usually have the best interests of the patient at heart; however, their advice may sometimes be misguided. We often ask patients if the information they are working from came from family, friends, or medical professionals.

This section deals with one's will and the will of others, including that of medical professionals. Your will may take a backseat to the will of family, friends, baby, and the medical system, and at times you might feel lost in the shuffle. Many pregnant women experience a decrease in their self-esteem because they just do not feel like themselves and things are happening to their bodies that are at times out of their control. When a Knight of the Belly tells of horrific birthing experiences, they can take an already frightened and vulnerable patient and scare the amniotic fluid right out of her. If you are a pregnant damsel in distress and have been taken on by a Knight of the Belly, remember that their cause is noble and true, but the information may be a little biased. The Knight is looking for a cause, and your pregnancy makes the Knight feel needed.

4. Honor Thy Family; Stay Connected

The divorce rate in 2006 was 3.6/1,000 people (CDC, 2006). What becomes lost in the statistics is the fact that divorce affects both parents and children. Divorce has an obvious influence during pregnancy, and pregnancy can even be the cause of some divorces in this country. The top ten reasons for divorce in 2005 are listed below.

- Husband had an affair
- Physical or mental abuse
- Boredom
- Lack of sex
- Financial disagreements
- Alcohol and drug abuse

- Debt
- Careers take priority over family
- Hobbies
- Wife had an affair

Some of the items on the list have to do with sexuality and personal survival. During pregnancy, both of these issues tend to be on high alert. There are also issues of codependency, poor boundaries, jealousy, and intimacy for pregnant women. To love and be loved is a basic requirement for human beings. When a woman learns she is pregnant, she becomes aware of the archetypes of Father, Mother, and, unfortunately, the Divorced Parent. It is through self-love and family support that women are able to make a healthy connection to the power of the Mother.

K. L. was a thirty-five-year-old woman who had recently moved into the Tucson area and just discovered she was pregnant. She and the father of the baby were not married, but they had a solid relationship and plans for marriage in the future. In the beginning of the pregnancy he attended her doctor visits and was actively involved with asking questions. Into the second trimester, however, I noticed that he had stopped coming to the visits. I did not think this abnormal since men do not always come to the prenatal visits.

On one particular antepartum visit, I remember seeing K. L. looking relatively somber. She explained that she had just left her job for employment with one of her prior competitors for a larger salary. This was not the explanation I had expected, since it seemed like a relatively good piece of information. The patient was nervous about taking this new position because she was going to be delivering in a few months and when she interviewed (weeks ago) she failed to mention to them that she was pregnant. It was apparent that she was dealing with anxiety, guilt, and fear at the same time. She left the office feeling a bit better but still conflicted.

Upon her return in three weeks she was very upset and tearful. She explained that her fiancé had recently told her that he no longer wanted to be part of the relationship and that he had no plans of participating in raising their baby. She had no idea what she was going to do or how she was going to care for this baby alone and with a new job. She stated that this recent breakup had made her relive some of her issues with her own father who had left the family when she was young. In looking at her situation, I felt it would be helpful if she could tap into the Maternal archetype to help her connect with a group outside of herself. Her mother was deceased, but she did have a sister, so I encouraged her to call her sister to see if she would help her as a labor coach.

At the next visit, K. L. brought her older sister, and every visit after that her sister was by her side, nurturing and caring for her. This nurturing provided by the sister filled a maternal gap that the patient had in her pregnancy, and it was this link that allowed K. L. to feel confident and stronger in her pregnancy and to feel more certain that she would soon become a wonderful mother. I am happy to report that K. L. delivered a beautiful little girl, went on to become one of the leading salespeople in her district, and her daughter has a loving, successful mother.

Obviously, the absent paternal figure, or Abandoning Father, affects an otherwise innocent child. This wound can be carried into the grown woman's pregnancy and cause a resurfacing of issues, especially if these issues have been suppressed. A broken home can lead to a broken patient. In the above example, the patient's failed relationship with her fiancé is merely an extension of her own imbalance. There are obviously many women who are single, pregnant, and loving the freedom of being on their own, but there is a stability that only the mother can bring to the pregnancy. This "mother" can be anyone from a sister, friend, or, ideally, a mother. According to Eastern Indian practice, the fourth chakra is the place of the heart and is synonymous with the sacrament of marriage—not necessarily the marriage of two people, but marriage of the external and internal worlds of the pregnant woman. This chakra can also represent the marriage of mother and baby. If the pregnant woman is not truly aligned and comfortable with the changes within her own body, then this imbalance can be symbolic of the pregnancy itself. Think of stabilization in the pregnancy coming about with an alignment of the woman with her family. If you are a new mother, try to connect with the maternal archetype that resonates best with you. If you are already a mother and pregnant with your second child, use this time to connect with the mother you want to become. If you and your mother have a relationship that is strained at best, try to think of what your part is in creating that relationship and hopefully repairing it in the future. In the story above, we saw a woman who was pushed into isolation, fear, and self-pity because of issues with abandonment and lack of a strong maternal presence. We also saw that she was brought back from her despair by the love and nurturing of her sister-mother figure. In order to try to connect with that emotional maternal archetype, we recommend trying some of the practices below:

1. Listen to music that is emotionally meaningful to you.
2. Ask your partner to gently massage you or indulge in a prenatal massage.
3. Learn about deep breathing and incorporate yoga into your life.
4. Be mindful of things that you feel are beautiful.
5. When you close your eyes, focus on the cool color of green.
6. Try playing vibrational instruments such as singing bowls tuned to the note F.
7. Hug another person at least once a day.

5. Understand Your Voice; Avoid the Herd Mentality

There are special cases during one's pregnancy when myths and superstitions contribute to a woman metaphorically losing her voice; she may not feel there is anything she can say. She has to decide when to speak up or whether to become part of the herd. This feeling is similar to how many adolescents experience the power of peer pressure. During pregnancy you enter into a phase when you are literally caring for the life of another being. You may sometimes find that you have feelings you don't completely understand; sometimes you just *know* something. Have you heard of mother's intuition? Is it possible that mother's intuition is a connection that starts between you and your unborn baby, almost a blending of unconscious thought? You are constantly barraged with information and you are trying to make the right decisions for you and your baby. During this time, truth becomes muddled with myths that may not be yours and may push you into making decisions that are not yours.

Is your will different from that of your unborn child? I believe the two could be connected, and that the connection begins at the time of conception. Some of my patients claim that they have more feelings of intuition when they become pregnant, and that this feeling deepens after the birth of the child. Could there be some heightened awareness that comes from the increased hormones of pregnancy? Women often say they feel physically different during certain points of their menstrual cycle. Just take a look at the word *hysterectomy.* This is a combination of the Latin terms *hyster* or *huestra* (uterus) and *ectomy* (removal of). It should also be pointed out that the Latin word *huestra* is the root of the English word *hysteria.* The term *hysteria* can be traced back to ancient Egypt, where descriptions of disease are believed to be caused by a wandering uterus. The word *hysterectomy,* then, can be translated to mean the "removal of hysteria." It is not a stretch to point out that many people today feel that the uterus and pelvic organs are the cause of the cycling of woman's moods. You often see this attitude portrayed in films and on TV shows. I remember when I was a young man of about thirteen and my mother had a hysterectomy. She would take a small burgundy-colored pill (estrogen) every day and that made her feel better. Often, when we would have a disagreement, and she was angry with me, I would say, "Did you take your pill today?" The fact that even children are aware that hormonal imbalance can be responsible for a woman's moods testifies to the fact that we as a culture do not fully understand the complexity of being a woman.

Composer, artist, healer, and author Stephen Halpern has said, "If it is true that we are what we eat, it may just as accurately be said that you are what you listen to. IF you listen to advice that is patronizing and detrimental then you may become that which you hear. One should try to find themselves a place where they can go recharge. If that means meditation or listening to soothing music, or going for a nature walk, then you should make time."

The woman who is unable to speak up for herself may also have issues with her self-esteem and have a tendency toward feeling easily embarrassed; she may not speak her mind for fear of humiliation. This harkens to the issue of following mindlessly versus following your intuition. If you are a first-time mother it can be difficult to trust your instincts, but in most instances you most likely have an idea of what is right for you. If you have questions, you can always call your physician.

6. You're Expecting, So Expect Nothing

If you develop substantially unrealistic expectations regarding the future, which greatly exceed what you are actually able to accomplish, then you are setting yourself up for failure and disappointment, which in turn can lead to lower self-esteem.

Since the first day you found out about your pregnancy, an imprint was made of how your baby would behave, look, sleep, and walk. Unfortunately, the baby does not know that you have designs on how it is supposed to be—he or she hasn't read the book. We often feel as though babies should come with different owner's manuals and that these manuals should be delivered months before the baby. While it is important for you to have a vision for the future, we ask for a bit of flexibility, whether toward the pregnancy, the labor, or the baby. The point of settings one's expectations in line is to recognize potential illusions and to help you perceive any patterns that you might be following an illusion. Illusion is obviously something that is not reality, and this altered reality can make its way into your pregnancy, as seen by the multitude of myths and superstitions surrounding pregnancy.

So, you're expecting. The question is, what are you expecting?

We like surprises, but we also like to control our lives and surroundings. This is no more prevalent than in the ultrasound room, where over 95 percent of patients ask the technician to tell them the gender of their baby. We want to know so we can decorate the nursery in blue or pink. Already an illusion of what the child will look like and how it will behave is set up in the minds of the parents. With the advent of 3-D and 4-D ultrasounds, we can not only know the gender but we can obtain a lifelike picture of the baby's face; black-and-white, two-dimensional views have been replaced by caricatures in real time. Now couples can say even earlier that the baby has Daddy's nose or Mommy's lips or Uncle Hector's ears. All of these bits of knowledge help piece together a virtual picture of your baby.

The potential problem is that this need to know can become obsessive. We discussed earlier that amniocentesis for genetics is the only sure way to know the gender, but the test comes with a 1 in 200 chance of preterm delivery and probable fetal demise. Thankfully, none of our patients have had such a need to know that they would endanger their pregnancy in this way, and to the best of our knowledge there are no physicians out there who would perform this test based only on the parents' need to know.

If you know the gender of your baby around the eighteenth week, you have twenty-two weeks to continue to build the image of this child in your head. With excessive compulsion there comes obsession, and obsession creates an illusion. If the illusion does not coalesce into the reality, there is a potential for disappointment and upheaval; this may lead to postpartum blues or depression.

It is not only the expectations for the baby that can contribute to a depression, it is the mother's view of herself as a nurturing woman. We bring this up only to open a dialogue regarding postpartum and potential postpartum depression. Myths and superstitions in pregnancy can make a woman feel as though she did something wrong or did not do everything in her power to prevent something from happening. Either of these scenarios is not a good foundation from which to start raising your child. Being open to the changes of pregnancy and allowing your expectations to ebb and flow will keep you out of the trappings of potential illusion. The baby will be what the baby will be.

Think of this quotation by psychologist Rollo May: "We participate in the forming of the future by virtue of our capacity to conceive of and respond to new possibilities, and to bring them out of imagination and then in actuality." You can help form the future of your pregnancy, labor, delivery experience, and even postpartum, but you must be ready to respond to new possibilities. A woman whose family is pressuring her to have a natural birth experiences labor and decides that she would like an epidural. Should this deviation from her expected action make her feel shame and a sense of failure? It is during just this type of experience that the people around you should comfort and support your decision—even if your decision does not conform to certain cultural or familial myths.

It is with a dulled intuition that women enter into postpartum depression. Many women may feel hopeless and as though no one can ever understand what they are going through, when the reality is that postpartum depression is not rare and it is treatable. Occasionally, and in addition to therapy, we recommend that women journal, or write down their pregnant journey and the postpartum experience. This exercise can open doors to inner feelings and give you and your family a chance to see into your thoughts. Journaling daily can be an exercise in talking to your soul or that spiritual side of your character. In journaling or even writing a conversation to another person, you can release your expectations; expectations about the pregnancy and yourself. This allows you to address your fears and anxieties in hopes of getting them out and letting them go. The journey of writing and releasing may get you closer to the point where you can empower yourself and control your fears. Here are a couple quotes from notable individuals regarding the journey of writing for the soul.

"I merely took the energy it took to pout and wrote some blues" —Duke Ellington.

"Learn to get in touch with the silence within yourself and know that everything in life has a purpose"—Elizabeth Kübler-Ross.

7. Ask Questions: Explore, Educate, and Enjoy

What pregnant woman doesn't have questions?

One of the reasons for writing this book is to encourage women to ask more questions. How many times have you gone to your doctor's appointments and said that you had a bunch of questions but you forgot to write them down. Our suggestion would be ... to write them down.

Exploration of the stories and myths around you, in your culture, is one of the best ways to connect with your family and community. In many instances you might find that healthcare providers cannot always come up with a good answer, so this process is an education for everyone. Let's take, for instance, the issue of heartburn during pregnancy. Sometimes over-the-counter antacids like TUMS and Rolaids just don't cut the mustard ... bad analogy, but at least it's spicy. Some women will assume there is nothing they can do and will succumb to the lure of advertising; sometimes it's just easier to buy what is readily available than it is to ask questions. The sad thing is that TUMS and Rolaids may make the problem worse. If you don't ask the question about heartburn, your healthcare provider won't be able to enlighten you on the following facts:

- During pregnancy it is probably better to eat five to six small meals a day than two to three large meals. There is a sphincter muscle at the bottom of your esophagus that keeps acid and food from coming back up into your throat. The increased levels of progesterone created by the placenta relax this sphincter valve, which might mean that larger amounts of food could increase stomach pressure and result in gastroesophageal reflux disease, also know as GERD.
- Try to allow at least two hours between your last meal and bedtime. The worst thing you can do is eat a large meal, increase the pressure in your stomach, and then lie down.
- Chew, chew, chew your food. The more work you do with your teeth, the less work you have to do with your stomach. The more time your food spends in your mouth, the longer it is exposed to sali-

vary enzymes and the more it breaks down. The more broken-down the food is when it gets to your stomach, the less time it will have to spend in your stomach breaking down, and the less time in your stomach, the less acid you will need.

- Don't eat things that make you feel worse. Hey, Doc! It hurts when I do this. Then don't do that. If you find that there are certain foods that make your acid problems worse, then stay away from those foods.
- Sleep with the head of your bed elevated. Keep in mind that simply elevating your pillow may make the problem worse because you are flexing the neck and thus you might increase abdominal pressure. You want to place a few books under the headboard of the bed so that the entire bed is slightly angled. This angle will allow gravity to help you in your quest to vanquish heartburn.
- If you are not getting relief from the basics, and the TUMS and Rolaids are working for only an hour or two, then it might be of benefit to speak with your provider about a prescription drug that would provide relief.

All of this education could be done in a ten-minute visit and would be sorely missed if you had to suffer for another two weeks prior to your next visit.

Notes

1. *Oprah Winfrey* show, aired November 11, 2004. Produced by Dianne Atkinson Hudson.

2. W. H. Butler and P. J. Wiggelsworth, "The Effects of Aflatoxin B on the Pregnant Rat," *British Journal of Experimental Pathology* 47 (1966): 242.

3. J. S. Chapman, "The Relation between Auditory Stimulation of Short Gestation Infants and Their Gross Motor Limb Activity," doctoral diss., New York University, 1975.

4. S. Shahidulla and P. G. Hepper, "Hearing in the Fetus: Prenatal Detection of Deafness," *International Journal of Prenatal and Perinatal Studies* 4, nos. 3–4 (1992): 235.

Epilogue

Pregnancy is a journey, and while there may be maps, some roads are marked better than others. Family, friends, and even strangers will try to guide you throughout your journey, but only you can choose the path. Your destination is a safe and healthy delivery, bringing your baby home, watching him or her sleep. It is amazing that babies do not come with instruction manuals, somehow tagged to the placenta, or mailed from some secret location. Just as each baby is an individual, so is your pregnancy completely unique to you. Sure, there are certain universal things, like avoiding cigarettes, but some things considered taboo by some may be another's daily mantra.

Trying to distill the information you receive from friends and family is like drinking water from a fire hydrant: you swallow some, but most of it rushes around you. We hope that this book was able to answer some of the questions and turn down the flow of the fire hydrant. There are still many questions that need to be answered, and we will be here to address them when the time comes. The questions in this book and the stories told come from our patients, and we are truly indebted to them for their honesty. We experience such joy when we see these babies still within the confines of your belly; a belly we watch grow and develop from that cute little bump to that "big bag of hurt," as one of my patients called it right before her due date. There is something magnetic about your pregnant belly. There is something that connects us all, and something that takes us back to where it all began. The next time someone touches your belly, remember, they are not simply touching you, they are touching the future of humanity.

Hopefully they ask before they touch.

Index

263